108 Stories of Taijiquan Healing

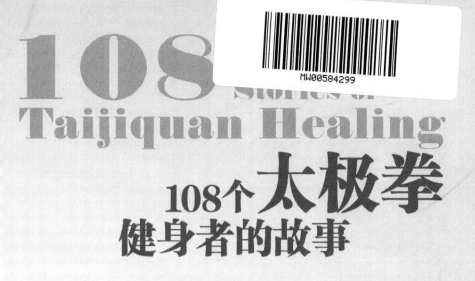

108个 太极拳
健身者的故事

Editor: Xinrong He，Steven Yang
编著：何新蓉，阳思达

Translated by Lu Dan，Rose Lo，Andrew Ensign，Sikai Yang
翻译：吕丹, Rose Lo, Andrew Ensign, 阳思凯

Proofreader: Yaolin Liu，Yulian Yang
审校：刘耀麟，阳喻联

Dixie W Publishing Corporation U.S.A.
美国南方出版社

108 个太极拳健身者的故事 / 何新蓉、阳思达 编著

Translated by Lu Dan，Rose Lo，Andrew Ensign，Sikai Yang
翻译：吕丹 , Rose Lo, Andrew Ensign, 阳思凯

Proofreader: Yaolin Liu Yulian Yang
审校：刘耀麟、阳喻联

108 Stories of Taijiquan Healing © 2022 by Xinrong He and Steven Yang

Published by
Dixie W Publishing Corporation
Montgomery, Alabama, U.S.A.
http://www.dixiewpublishing.com

本书由美国南方出版社出版
▪ 版权所有 侵权必究 ▪
2022 年 12 月 DWPC 第一版

开本：229mm × 152mm
字数：124 千字

Library of Congress Preassigned Control Number: 2022949235
美国国会图书馆预编目号码：2022949235
国际标准书号 ISBN-13: 978-1-68372-493-3

About the author 编著者简介

He Xinrong 何新蓉

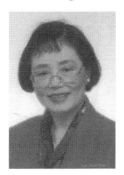

Editor, He Xinrong 编著者 何新蓉

He Xinrong: Doctor of Acupuncture and Oriental Medicine, Professor at the American Academy of Acupuncture and Oriental Medicine and Acupunctrist.Her publications are as follows:

(1) Yang-Style Taijiquan And Health Care, 1995, authors are she and her father as will as her husband; (2) Identify Diseases By Look At The ears, which won the "Golden Key Award"of 1995 National Book; (3) The Sorrows And Joys Under The Stars And Stripes Flag .2011; (4) Chinese-English Handbook for Seeing a Doctor in the USA. Oct. 2013; (5) Love Teachers.Published in June, 2021.

Her has obtained:

(1) Her Book 《Identify Desease by Examing Ears》 won the China National Book Golden Key Award in 1995; (2) Her paper

《Identify Desease by Examing Ears》. won the first prize of the second International Acupuncture Conference in Los Angeles in 1995

何新蓉：针灸和东方医学博士，美国中医学院教授，针灸师。发表作品如下：

(1)《杨式太极拳与保健》1995 年出版，作者是她和她的父亲何明以及她的丈夫刘耀麟；(2)《观耳识病》1994 年 9 月出版；(3)《星条旗帜下的悲欢离合》2011 年 4 月出版；(4)《英汉对照旅美就医手册》2013 年 10 月出版；(5)《吾爱吾师》2021 年 6 月出版。

获奖作品：

(1)《观耳识病》获得 1995 年中国国家图书金钥匙奖

(2) 论文《Identify Desease by Examing Ears》. 获得 1995 年洛杉矶第二届国际针灸大会一等奖

Steven Yang 阳思达

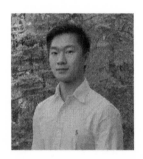

Editor, Steven Yang 编著者 阳思达

Steven Yang: Minnesota high school student. He has obtained:

(1) 2022 The MIT Agelab, OMEGA Scholarship; (2) 2022 U.S.A International "Star Leadership" program：1 st Place Star Leader Award; (3) 2022 Minnesota HOSA-Future Health Professionals Competition"The

Benefits of Taijiquan to Physical and Mental Health":1 st Place in Health Education; (4) TWIN CITIES INTERNATIONAL 2022 JBJJF JIU-JITSU CHAMPIONSHIP : Bronze Medal; (5) 2021 Minnesota Brazilian Jiu-Jitsu Competition: Gold Medal (Junior); (6) 2022, he published article about Taijiquan and health in the Minnesota newspaper "China Tribune".

阳思达：明尼苏达州高中生。曾获得：

(1) 2022 年麻省理工学院 Agelab，欧米茄奖学金；(2) 2022 年美国国际"明星领导力计划"中获"明星领袖奖"第一名；(3) 2022 年明尼苏达州 HOSA 美国未来卫生专业人才竞赛：《太极拳对身心健康的好处》获健康教育项目第一名；(4) 2022 双城国际 JBJJF 巴西柔术锦标赛：铜牌；(5) 2021 明尼苏达州巴西柔术比赛：金牌（青少年组）；(6) 2022 年，在明州华兴报发表太极拳与健康有关文章。

Dedicate this book
to
Mr. He Ming, and
Friends who love Taijiquan.

谨以此书献给

何明老先生及

爱好太极拳的朋友们

Two Poems For Taijiquan 太极拳诗二首

By He Ming 何明

1. One

Movement rests in Taiji, 动在太极，

harmonizing Qi and blood, 调和气血。

Still and tranquil, 静而安宁，

following the breath to refresh the spirit. 随息养神。

Enjoyment erases our burdens, 乐以忘忧，

in good spirits and relaxed nature. 怡情悦性。

Long and healthy life, 寿世且康，

preciousness lies in perseverance. 贵在有恒。

2. Two

Form is pliant as swishing willows, 形柔轻拂柳，

Mind-set, a serene pine, enter deep meditation, 意静松入禅。

Happy and contented, Qi harmoniously combines, 怡然气配合，

Oblivious and withdrawn from the human realm. 忘却在人间。

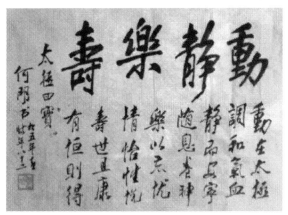

Preface 前言

By Dr. Xinrong He

In today's fast-paced society, stroke, coronary heart disease, hypertension, hyperlipidemia, diabetes, anxiety, depression, and even cancer have become common and frequently occurring diseases. During the COVID-19 pandemic around the world, the number of people with anxiety disorders has skyrocketed.

Anxiety disorders are the most common mental illness in the United States, affecting 40 million Americans aged 18 and older [1].

On December 23, 2020, the State Council Information Office of China held a press conference to introduce the "Report on Nutrition and Chronic Disease Status of Chinese Residents". 19 years of data show that the prevalence of anxiety disorders reached 4.98%. (As many as 67 million based on a population of 1.4 billion.)

How can you keep yourself physically and mentally healthy? Especially, when COVID-19 is rampantly spreading around the world, how can we strengthen our immune system and reduce anxiety? How can the elderly maintain a healthy quality of life?

The author strongly recommends practicing Taijiquan to strengthen your physical and mental health, reduce anxiety, and improve your quality of life.

Taijiquan has a history of hundreds of years in China, and it is a precious heritage of Chinese traditional martial arts. The ancient Taijiquan is based on the theory of Yin and Yang of Taiji. It can connect the meridians, tune the virtual and real, and adjust the five zang organs (hear, liver, spleen, kidney). It is a soft, relaxed, internal and external combination, dynamic and static combination of the whole body movement. It is similar to the quiet and inaction of Taoism, the four empty principles of Buddhism, and the middle mean doctrine of Confucianism, which is the way to cultivate the mind and cultivate nature. They are all different approaches to achieving equally satisfactory results.

Taijiquan is also a fitness technique that integrates Qigong, philosophy, meditation, culture, and martial arts. It is one of the best styles that are most suitable for everyone's fitness and can also improve one's essence Qi spirit. Taijiquan uses the waist as the axis to drive the whole body to rotate so that the muscles, bones and joints of the whole body can be exercised, which has a good effect on relieving pain. Taijiquan is one of the best martial arts with scientific principles.

Practicing Taijiquan, like another aerobic exercise, can release beta-endorphins. Scientists point out that endorphins can release emotional elements in the brain, making people feel happy and full of vitality, thereby improving mental states.

Thus, practicing Taijiquan will have immeasurable value on public health and mental health.

The study by the University of Applied Sciences in Coburg, Germany found that salivary cortisol (stress hormone) was significantly reduced after 18 weeks of Taijiquan practice, and mental stress was also significantly reduced during follow-up [2].

A study by the University of Queensland in Australia showed that after 6 months of Taijiquan intervention, anxiety and stress were significantly improved, and mental and heart health had also improved [3].

The graduate school of Nara Women's University, Japan, studied the changes in the brain waves of Taijiquan practitioners: the high anxiety group was in a state of moderate alertness with the increase of $\alpha 1$, $\alpha 2$, and $\beta 1$ rhythms during the completion of Taijiquan exercise and recovery; their mood was calm and the body and mind were relaxed. These participants were focused and entered a low anxiety state. The anxiety level of the subjects in the low anxiety group was reduced to the lowest level through Taijiquan exercise, and it was shown that their mental states were not easily affected by external conditions and stress [4].

In April 2022, Singapore Longitudinal Ageing Study on the Association of Taijiquan Exercise with Physical and Neurocognitive Function, Frailty, Quality of Life, and Mortality in the Elderly was published. The results show that regular Taijiquan exercise can improve the quality of life (QOL) and reduce the prevalence of mental and physical ailments [5].

Scientists in Europe have conducted a 10-week experimental study on people aged 60-78 during the COVID-19 pandemic. This study group learned Taijiquan twice a week, 60 minutes each time. The results of the study found that Taijiquan is an effective intervention method to improve the emotional state, cognition, and physical functions of the elderly [6].

In July 2002, Time Magazine compared the ancient Chinese Taijiquan movement to the perfect movement. In 2020, the Beijing Administration of Traditional Chinese Medicine has included Taijiquan and Baduanjin in the citywide COVID-19 prevention plan.

The author participated in the first Harvard Medical Qigong Tai Chi Forum in 2018 hosted by the American Chinese Medicine Association (ATCMA). More than 200 attendees came from all over the world,including many Tai Chi experts and Dr.He Deguang,the director of the American Tai Chi Qigong Committee.Special guest speakers included: Harvard University's famous Professor Peter WAYNE,Professor Herbert Benson, Professor Jin Guanyuan and Professor Liu Tianjun (China), et al.

They cited a lot of scientific data and examples proving that Tai Chi is the perfect exercise, which is very beneficial to physical and mental health!

The father of this book's chief editor, Mr. He Ming, suffered from hemoptysis due to tuberculosis in 1933. There was no cure at that time, so he learned Taijiquan with the curator of Shaoxing martial arts Mr. Zeng Shouchang, (friend of Yang Chengfu, Master of Yang Style Taijiquan), and he recovered from the disease years later.

After Dr. He's father benefited from it, he began to share it with others and voluntarily spread Taijiquan for 67 years, gaining tens of thousands of disciples. He also won the Taijiquan Championship at The Whampoa Military Academy.

Taijiquan helped Mr. He Ming keep his legs and feet flexible, and at the age of nearly 80, he climbed Mount Emei and descended into the Gobi Desert in Xinjiang. At the age of 87, he still walk in Yellowstone National Park and hiked in the 3713-meter-high Rocky Mountain National Park in the United States. He said while he is alive, he'll never stop teaching Taijiquan. He wanted to teach Taijiquan for the rest of his life until he saw God. He wishes people all over the world to learn Taijiquan to enhance their physical and mental health!

Thirty years ago, my father, my husband, and I wrote the book "Yang Style Taijiquan and Health Care," which has been printed many times to illustrate the need for Taijiquan. Although my father has passed away now, we have inherited his legacy and have been teaching Taijiquan for more than40 years.

After arriving in the USA, we have continued to promote Taijiquan for 27 years, with thousands of students. We are happy to see that not only Chinese people, practice Taijiquan, foreigners love Taijiquan, also, and they have a very high opinion of Taijiquan. They say Taijiquan has changed their lives.

Young student Steven Yang, one of the editors of this book, started to teach Taijiquan for free in high schools and nursing homes, as well as the community after learning Taijiquan from me. I am delighted to see that there are successors in spreading Taijiquan.

The book 《108 Stories of Taijiquan Healing》 is not about teaching and practicing Taijiquan, but rather stories told by Chinese and foreign friends about the benefits of practicing: anxiety patients feel calm; patients suffering from depression experience relief; cancer patients feel enhanced immunity and self-healing power, so that they can coexist with cancer for many years; the sequelae of the drug addicts disappear, and they are able to work energetically; the overweight become slender; kidney functions return to normal after practicing Taijiquan for those with renal insufficiency. After a car accident, She was unable to work for 20 years due to muscle pain, and she is able to work. There are many such examples in this book.

It is the hope of the author that this book can be shared with friends and families, and that people can participate in the practice of Taijiquan to gain health and happiness! Then the author's original intention has been achieved.

在当代竟争激烈的社会中，由于工作紧张，脑中风、冠心病、高血压、高血脂、糖尿病、焦虑症、抑郁症、甚至癌症已成了常见病、多发病。在全世界处于新冠疫情期间，焦虑症的患者更是猛增。

在美国，焦虑症是最常见的精神疾病，影响了年龄在 18 岁及以上的四千万美国成年人 [1]。

2020 年 12 月 23 日，国务院新闻办召开新闻发布会，介绍《中国居民营养与慢性病状况报告》的有关情况。19 年数据显示，焦虑障碍的患病率达到 4.98%。（以 14 亿人口计算多达 6 千 7 百多万。）

怎样让自己身心健康？尤其是当前冠状肺炎在全球疯狂蔓延之际，如何增强自己的免疫力与治愈率？减少焦虑症？老年人怎样才能保持有质量的生活呢？

笔者强烈推荐练习太极拳来帮助你身心健康，减少焦虑症，乐观向上！

太极拳在中國已有几百年历史，是中华民族传统武术的珍贵遗产。古老的太极拳以太极的阴阳学说为理论依据，可以通经络、调虚实、调五脏，是一种柔和、放松、内外结合、动静结合的全身运动。它与道教的清静无为，佛教的四大皆空，儒家的中庸之道等异曲同工，是修心养性之道。

太极拳是将气功、武术、哲学、医学、文化、技击等融为一体的健身拳术，能健身、益智、防病、治病，增强人的精气神。太极拳以腰为轴，带动全身，让周身肌肉、筋骨、关节得到锻炼，对减轻身体疼痛有很好的作用。太极拳是体育运动中最合乎健身，具有科学原理的优秀武术之一。

练太极拳和其它有氧运动一样，可以释放 β-内啡肽，科学家指出，内啡肽（endorphins）能让大脑释放情绪元素，使人感到快乐、幸福和充满活力，从而改善不良的心理状态。

因此，练太极拳对公众健康和心理健康有着不可估量的价值。

德国科堡应用科学大学的研究发现：练习太极拳18周后唾液皮质醇（压力荷尔蒙）显著降低，随访中也发现精神压力显著下降[2]。

澳大利亚昆士兰大学研究显示：练习太极拳6个月后，焦虑和压力显着改善，还增加了心理和心脏健康[3]。

日本国立奈良女子大学研究生院研究练习太极拳对脑电波的变化：高焦虑组在完成太极拳运动和恢复期间，随着 α_1，α_2，β_1 节律的增加，身体处于中度警觉状态，并且心情平静，身心放松，注意力集中，进入低焦虑状态；原本处于低焦虑组受试者的焦虑水平，通过太极拳运动降至最低水平，并不容易受到外部条件和压力等因素的影响[4]。

2022年4月新加坡纵向老龄化研究项目发表了太极运动与老年

人身体和神经认知功能、虚弱、生活质量和死亡率的关系。其结果表明：经常性的太极拳锻炼，可以提高生活质量 (QOL)，患病率降低[5]。

欧洲的科学家在 covid-19 大流行期间，对 60-78 岁的老年人，进行了 10 个星期实验研究。即每星期学习 2 次太极拳，每次 60 分钟。研究结果发现：太极拳是一种有效的干预手段，太极拳可以改善老年人的情绪状态、认知和身体功能[6]。

2002 年 7 月美国《时代周刊》将中国古老的太极拳运动比喻为完美运动。2020 年，北京中医药管理局已经将太极拳，八段锦列入了防治新冠肺炎方案中。

笔者曾参加由全美中医药学会（ATCMA）主办的 2018 年首届哈佛大学医学气功太极论坛。与会者 200 多人，来自世界各地。有许多太极专家，还有美国太极气功委员会主任贺德广，及特邀讲员：哈佛大学著名的彼得·韦恩教授 [Prof. Peter WAYNE, Ph.D.]，赫波特 本森教授 [Prof. Herbert Benson, M.D.]，美国的金观源教授 [Prof. Guanyuan JIN] 北京的刘天君教授 [Prof. Tianjun LIU] 等。他们用大量的科学数据及实例表明太极拳是完美的运动，极有利于心身健康！

本文作者的父亲何明老先生，1933 年因肺结核咯血，当时无药可治，随绍兴国术馆长曾寿昌先生（杨氏太极拳大师杨澄甫的好友）学习太极拳后，他的疾病无药自愈。

父亲练太极拳获益后，开始与人分享，义务传播太极拳 67 年，弟子数万。何明老先生还曾在黄埔军校获得太极拳冠军。太极拳让他腿脚灵活，近 80 高龄还可以上登峨眉山，下入新疆戈壁滩。87 岁时还能游走在美国黄石公园及 3713 米高的落基山国家公园。他表示生命不息，教拳不已。要一生教太极拳直到见上帝！他愿天下的人学习太极拳，获得身心健康！

30 年前，我与父亲、及我的先生曾写过《杨式太极拳与医疗保健》一书，此书已多次印刷，说明人们需要太极拳。如今父亲虽已远离人世，但是我们继承父亲的遗志，40 多年来一直坚持不懈地教太极拳。到美国后继续推广太极拳已经 27 年，学生数千。我们高兴地看到不仅国人，就是外国人同样热爱太极拳，他们对太极拳的评价极高，认为太极拳改变了他们的生活。编著者之一的阳思达同学，在学完太极拳后，便开始在社区、学校和养老院免费教太极拳，欣喜地看到传播太极拳后继有人。

本书《108 个太极拳健身者的故事》，其特点是中外拳友自己讲述练习太极拳后给自身的健康带来的好处：焦虑症患者心情平静了；抑郁症病人症状减轻，不再厌世；癌症病人增强了免疫力和自愈力，多年来能与癌共存；戒毒者后遗症消失，能够精力充沛去工作；体重超高者变苗条了；肾功能不全者练拳后肾功能恢复了正常；车祸后因肌肉疼痛 20 年不能工作者，疼痛大减，重新开始工作 ....。书中诸如此类的实例很多。

愿此书能够与更多的朋友与家人分享！参与修练太极拳，从而获得健康、快乐！则作者初衷达到。

Table of Content 目录

XVI

XVIII

A Inspiring stories
启发人的故事

1. Taijiquan and I 太极拳和我

By Lin Yee Chen MD

Taijiquan is a traditional Chinese martial art. Ever since I was a child, I had a strong desire to learn Taijiquan, but I never found the opportunity.

In 2019, due to health reasons, I strengthened my determination to learn Taijiquan and finally found two teachers. One teacher taught Yang style Taijiquan (24 styles and 118 styles), and the other taught Chen style Taijiquan (old style) and Baduanjin.

Since 2020, my exercise routine is to practice Yang Style Taijiquan (24 Forms) and Baduanjin every morning, and Chen Style Taijiquan or Yang Style Taijiquan (118 Forms) in the afternoon. In the past three years, I have never missed a day of practice.

I actively practice Taijiquan and Qigong because of the various benefits they bring to me. Below I will describe my association with Taijiquan from two different viewpoints.

First, as a cardiologist, practicing Taijiquan has benefitted me a lot. Medical research has shown that Taijiquan and Qigong not only help reduce risk factors for heart disease (high blood pressure, high cholesterol, etc.), but also help improve balance and coordination, prevent falls, enhance cognitive ability, and prevent dementia. Not only that, Taijiquan and Qigong can also reduce mental stress, regulate emotions, and prevent depression and anxiety.

Secondly, Taijiquan is one of the cultural heritage of the Chinese nation. As a Chinese person, preserving this priceless legacy is a top priority. Taijiquan contains profound philosophical concepts, such as the Taoism concept of harmony between yin and yang; it teaches us many principles of living as well as doing things, such as coming and going, pushing and pulling, etc.

Learning is a journey of life, "a journey of a thousand miles begins with a single step." Learning Taijiquan is no exception. I plan to continue learning other traditional styles of Taijiquan, and make it my lifelong ambition to learn Taijiquan.

Note: Doctor Chen is currently the Director of Lillehei Heart Institute at the University of Minnesota. He is very busy, but he still practices Taijiquan every day.

太极拳是中国传统武术之一。从小我有极强意愿学太极拳，但一直没找到机会。

2019 年，由于健康原因，我坚定了学太极拳的决心，于是找到两位老师，一位老师教导杨氏太极拳（24 式及 118 式），另一位老师教导陈氏太极拳（老架一路）及八段锦。

从 2020 年至今，我运动的常规是每天清晨练 24 式太极拳与八段锦，下午便练陈氏太极拳或者杨氏太极拳（118 式）。这三年以来，我从未错过一天的练习。

我之所以积极练习太极拳和气功是因为其带来各种各样的益处。以下我将从两个不同的身份描述太极拳与我的关联。

首先，对我作为一名心脏科专家而言，太极拳大有裨益。医学研究显示，太极拳和气功不但利于降低心脏疾病危险因素（高血压，高胆固醇等），它还利于提高平衡和协调能力，防止摔倒，加强认知能力及预防失智症。不仅如此，太极拳和气功也可减轻精神压力、调节情绪、预防抑郁与焦虑症。

其次，对我身为一位中国人而言，太极拳为中华民族文明遗产之一。作为一位中国人，保留该无价之宝的遗产是重中之重。太极拳蕴含深刻哲学理念，例如道教的阴阳概念；教导我们许多做人原则，以及它教给我们许多生活和做事的原则，如来与往、推与拉等。

学习是人生旅途，千里之行，始於足下。学太极拳也不例外。新冠疫情过去后，我打算继续学其他传统太极拳流派，将学习太极拳作为我毕生之志。

注：曾大夫现任明尼苏达大学心脏科移植研究所的主任。该研究所为 Lillehei Heart Institute。他非常忙，但是依然每天坚持练习太极拳。

2. Grow with Taijiquan 与太极拳共同成长

By Steven Yang

Indifference is the bane that threatens progress and potential. Every day, we are surrounded by tragedies from every corner of the globe. Although we feel sympathy and indignation, we believe these events are outside our control; we learn to live on. We grow accustomed to the cruel realities of the world and push them into the recesses of our minds, believing someone else will solve them sooner or later The same mentality took root in my mind until last summer when I read the news of a brutal racial attack nearby: A ten-year-old Asian boy was beaten and called racial slurs for supposedly spreading COVID. Initially, my habitual indifference prevented me from taking action. But as time moved on and similar events took place all around me, I began to blame those who had authority but were mute toward injustice. Eventually, however, my anger crept into shame as I questioned myself: would I've stood up? Would my actions even change anything? Moreover, would I be saved if I were attacked? My hesitancy made me uneasy. Convinced that someone better would always exist, I was trapped in a cycle of hypocrisy, hating inaction but never standing up to help.Grow with Taijiquan

Six years ago, I had the opportunity to begin studying under Dr. He. Throughout the years, I slowly began to view Taijiquan as a way to foster holistic wellness and understanding between cultures. Not only can it help Americans understand Chinese culture, but it is also a gentle and effective exercise to improve the mental and physical health of busy students. I believe that when people are physically and mentally healthy, that is when true understanding starts. Hatred and hostility can be slowly transformed into love and appreciation for the differences between cultures.

At the start of my first Taijiquan class, a woman slowly stepped through the door. I greeted the old woman but was met by skeptical eyes. Without much introduction, the woman asked me about how Taijiquan could improve her condition. The majority of her back was immobilized after a horrific fall, causing most daily tasks to become insurmountable. I gave her my best answers but she still needed more convincing. Her disbelief chipped at my conviction for the entire session, but I refused to see this project amount to nothing. The following week, the woman stepped through the door again. She was no longer resistant, but her air of skepticism remained. I knew the benefits of Taijiquan would be invaluable to her, and we just needed persistence.

Weeks passed and I greeted more and more unfamiliar faces each session. After seeing the effects of Taijiquan and her persistence, the woman invited her friends who suffered from similar conditions. I never expected my impact to reach so many people. And speaking of the woman, her shell finally cracked. Her eyes glistened with resilience and her steps were budding with vitality. These changes mirrored my own journey. I wasn't the most talented teacher or practitioner, but with passion and enthusiasm, we explored the intricacies of the art together while enjoying its benefits. Although I cannot control the outcomes, the warmth, smiles, and stories of progress I receive in return fuel my confidence and determination to continue contributing in any way I can.

Teaching Taijiquan pushed me to fulfill my potential. I learned that anyone can create positive change from a small step forward. And because of that, I could never settle for indifference again.

Grow with Taijiquan !

冷漠是阻碍人们自我反省和社会文明进步的麻醉剂。每一天，我们都被来自全球每个角落的悲剧所包围。虽然我们感到同情和愤慨，但我们相信这些事件不是我们所能控制的；我们学会了与冷漠共存。我们逐渐习惯了世界上残酷的现实，并熟视无睹，相信别人迟早会解决这些问题。

直到去年夏天，当我读到我们居住的小区附近发生种族袭击的新闻：一名10岁的亚裔男孩被人无故殴打，并实施种族歧视性辱骂他是COVID-19的传播者。最初，习惯性的冷漠让我无动于衷。随着时间的推移，当身边不断有同样的事发生的时候，我又会生出一股愤怒，我指责那些有权利却对不公正保持沉默的人；随后又生出一些侥幸，希望有更好的人能处理好这些事情。然而，有一种叫良知的东西让我的缄默变成了羞愧，我问自己：如果这件事发生在我面前，我会站出来吗？甚至这样的事就发生在自己身上，我会得救吗？我能期待别人做什么？于是我陷入了虚伪的怪圈，讨厌别人的无所作为，自己却不为改变这种不公正的事情做出努力。

六年前，一个偶然的机会我跟随何博士学习太极拳，经过六年的学习，我逐渐认识到太极拳不仅可以增加美国人对了解中国传统文化的兴趣，而且是一种可改善学习繁忙的学生身心健康的、温和有效的锻炼方式。我相信，当人的身体和心理都健康时，就是人们相互理解的开始，仇恨和敌意就会慢慢转变为爱和欣赏，相互包容不同文化之间的差异。

当我的第一堂公益太极拳课堂开始时，一位老妇人慢慢地踏入了教室。我向那位驼背的老妇人打了个招呼，但得到的却是怀疑的目光。没有太多介绍，她就问我太极如何能改善她的背痛状况。她在一次可怕的摔倒后，背部多处受伤，导致大多数日常生活都变得难以完成。我尽力给她解释了太极拳的益处，虽然她质疑的态度在整个交流中削弱了我的信念，但是我坚持教授她练习太极拳。接下来的一个星期，她又一次走进教室。她不再固执，但仍然带着怀疑的神情。我知道太极对她的好处是无价的，我鼓励并带领她坚持练习。

几个星期过去了，逐渐看到练习太极拳的效果后，她带来了她的朋友，并且乐于面对新来的人讲述自己身体的变化。现在每次教授太极拳课堂我都要和越来越多的陌生面孔打招呼，我从没想过太极拳会影响到这么多人。我清楚地了解自己不是最好的太极拳老师或实践者，但我对练习太极拳充满着激情和爱。当我与我的太极拳学员们一起探索这种东方武术的复杂性的同时，也享受它带来的好处。

虽然我无法预测未来的困境，但我收到太极拳学员们的温暖、微笑和进步的故事反过来增添了我的信心和决心，让我继续尽我所能为社会做出贡献。

教太极拳激发了我的潜能，我明白了任何人都可以从一个小小的"我再也不会冷漠"中创造积极的改变，从而提高人与人之间的信任度。

我与太极拳共同成长！

3. My Experience with Taijiquan
我练太极拳的经验

Esther Peralez Ph.D 博士

My experience with Taijiquan began in approximately 1995. I was seeing Dr. He at the time for acupuncture. Also, I decided to start working on my doctorate.

I worked at the University of Minnesota, in a high demanding job holding the post of Departmental Director, Student and Instructional Support Services General College. At this time I hold the post of Special Assistant to Vice President of Student Development & Athletics

The job; beginning of menopause; and the doctorate expectations resulted in me becoming more anxious, forgetful, and highly stressed out. It was during my doctoral written exam that I finally realized that I needed help. My husband, who had done acupuncture in the past, suggested I try it.

Dr. He was recommended to me. After a couple of sessions, I was so impressed by Dr. He's results. She seemed to know my symptoms before I even described them and I felt changes within days. Shortly after meeting with her for acupuncture, she suggested I enroll in her Taijiquan class. I was assured that Taijiquan would complement the acupuncture treatments and also help with my anxiety, mood, memory and sleep.

Also, I decided to start working on. I started the class and was a little nervous about not knowing any of the movements. The first couple of classes were stressful because I was concentrating too much on how to correctly do the movements. While I was supposed to concentrate on my breathing and body sensations, I found myself holding my breath and having jerky body motions. Soon, I gained confidence in my movements and breathing. All of a sudden, I would forget everything around me and the focus was on my breathing and body. It truly made me relaxed and calm. I quickly realized the benefits of Taijiquan, including better balance.

Because of the calming, relaxing feel experienced during Taijiquan, I practiced it faithfully beyond the class time and after my class enrollment ended. Dr. He was so committed to and believed in the benefits of Taijiquan, that she allowed her former students to attend her current classes for a refresher. I took advantage of that benefit a number of times. She also encouraged us to practice in nature to further feel the calming effects. Once a month on Sunday, she invited anyone who wanted to attend to join her and her family in a Taijiquan exercise in the park. She was right. The outdoor experience was wonderful.

On a personal note, she invited my husband and me to join her on a trip to China for her son's wedding. That was the most wonderful experience. However, the most memorable moment was when she and her siblings showed us where her father, a Taijiquan master, used to practice Taijiquan. They did a routine for us at that same exact spot(Shaoxing). For me, it made me truly appreciate how long Taijiquan had been around but also to be associated with people who had practiced it all their lives and were thriving because of it. It was so meaningful.

I moved out of Minnesota in 2007. While I immediately began acupuncture again, I only practiced Taijiquan at home, by myself. I was in another high demanding job. Employment at The City College of New York (CCNY) holds the post of Served as President's designee to undergraduate and student governments. hold the post of Served as a member of the President's Council and the President's Cabinet that address. I practiced Taijiquan to help with my anxiety, moods, memory, stress, sleep, energy and overall health. I survived that very demanding job, too.

In 2012, I moved back to Minnesota and lived in Winona. While there, I was diagnosed with arthritis of my hips. To help with the inflammation, I started acupuncture but also started reading to find the best exercise to deal with arthritis. Taijiquan was listed because of its low impact on your bones. Once again, I practiced at home to ensure I kept my balance and flexibility. It definitely made a difference.

In 2018, my husband and I retired and moved to Pennsylvania. Again, I began acupuncture but this time I signed up for a Taijiquan class when the facilities started opening again after COVID. I enrolled in it for a year. During that time, I also swam and practiced Taijiquan in the water. Because swimming and Taijiquan have a low impact on your bones, my mind and body felt good when I got out of the pool.

The current gym I joined has Taijiquan classes. I continue to swim and plan on enrolling in the next session in the fall. I am grateful to Dr. He for encouraging me to enroll in her Taijiquan class many years ago. The practice has definitely added to my physical and mental health and sustained my ability to do all that I do as I age.

Taijiquan has become part of my life and my quality of life is good because of it.

我打太极拳的经历大约开始于 1995 年。我当时正在看何医生，她是针灸师。此外，我还决定开始攻读我的博士学位。

我在明尼苏达大学工作，是一份要求很高的工作。曾担任学生和教学支持服务综合学院的系主任。后担任学生发展与体育副校长的特别助理。

这份工作和更年期的开始以及对博士学位的期望，让我变得更加焦虑、健忘和高度紧张。在我的博士论文准备中，我于是意识到我需要帮助。我丈夫过去做过针灸，建议我试试。

我被推荐给了何医生。经过几次治疗后，我对何医生的治疗结果感到如此的震惊。她似乎在我描述症状之前就知道我的状况，几天后我就感到了变化。在和她做针灸治疗后不久，她建议我去参加她的太极拳课。我确信，太极拳可以补充针灸治疗，也有助于缓解我的焦虑、改善情绪和记忆以及睡眠。

我决定开始上太极拳课。因为不知道任何一个动作而有点紧张，前几节课的压力很大，因为我太专注如何正确地做这些动作了。当我集中精力在我的呼吸和身体感觉时，我发现我对自己的动作和呼吸有了信心。突然之间，我会忘记我周围的一切，重点放了在我的呼吸和身体，这真的让我放松和平静。我很快就意识到了太极拳的好处，包括更好的平衡性。

由于太极拳过程中经历的平静、放松的感觉，我在上课时间和课后坚持了练习。何医生如此致力于太极拳并相信太极拳的好处，她允许她以前的学生参加她现在的课程来复习。我多次利用这一好处。她还鼓励我们在大自然中练习，以进一步感受到平静的效果。每月一次的星期天，她邀请任何想参加的人加入她和她的家人在公园参加太极拳运动。她是对的。户外活动的体验非常棒。

何医生还邀请我和丈夫一起去中国参加了她儿子的婚礼，那是最美妙的经历。然而，最难忘的时刻是她和她的兄弟姐妹告诉我们，她的父亲，一位太极拳大师—过去开始练习太极拳的地方（绍兴）。在同一地点他们为我们演示了一套太极拳。对我来说，它让我真正体会太极拳的悠久历史，也让我与那些一生都在练习太极拳，并因此而茁壮成长的人联系在了一起。它是如此地有意义！

2007年，我搬出了明尼苏达州。在家里练习太极拳。我在做另一份要求很高的工作，在纽约城市学院工作。被任命做本科生和学生会的校长指定行政官员，还担任校长理事会和内阁的成员。所以我练习了太极拳来帮助我缓解焦虑、情绪、压力、帮助睡眠、精力和整体健康。我也在那份非常苛刻的工作中挺了下来。

2012 年，我搬回了明尼苏达州，住在威诺纳。在那里，我被诊断出患有臀部关节炎。为了帮助缓解炎症，我开始针灸，但也开始阅读，寻找治疗关节炎的最佳运动。太极拳被列入名单是因为它对骨骼的冲击力很小。再一次，我在家里练习，以确保我保持平衡和灵活性。这确实会有所不同。

2018 年，我和丈夫退休后搬到了宾夕法尼亚州。我又开始针灸，但这一次我报名参加了一个太极拳课，在新冠肺炎后，运动设施又开始开放。我注册了一年，在那段时间里，我在水里游泳和练习太极拳。因为游泳和太极拳对骨骼的冲击力很小，所以当我走出游泳池时，我的身心都感觉很好。

我现在加入的健身房里有太极拳课。我继续游泳，并计划报名参加秋季的下一节课程。我很感谢何博士。她多年前鼓励我参加她的太极拳课。这种练习无疑增加了我的身心健康，并维持了我随着年龄的增长，在年老时能够继续做我所要做的一切。

太极拳已经成为我生活的一部分，我的生活质量也因此变得很好。

4. The Experience of Practicing Taijiquan
练太极拳的心得

By Kuo Mama

When I was a student, I often read about Taijiquan and Qigong in articles and magazines, but I didn't care. For me, it was just a term in Chinese culture that held no relevancy .

After entering the workforce, for a while, like most people, I was obsessed with Jin Yong's martial arts novels. Stories such as "Legend of the Dragonslayer Sword（a Chinese movie）", in which Zhang Sanfeng, the head of the Wudang order, learned Taijiquan and Taijijian after 18 months of intense study, and taught them to the Mingjiao order called Wuji, or the one about Fang Dongbai, the eight-armed legend who used his Taijiquan to beat away the head of the four elders of the bandit gang and brought peace to his homeland embedded Taijiquan deeply in my mind ever since.

After crossing the ocean to the United States, I had the opportunity to study Traditional Chinese Medicine in the College of Traditional Chinese Medicine. As an elective course, I chose to learn Taijiquan. Fortunately, we were taught Taijiquan by Dr. He Xinrong, who comes from a family of Taijiquan. Dr. He was very patient and taught us every move, step by step. She taught us very carefully, and we also learned every move carefully. In this way, teachers and students worked together to learn the 24 forms of style Taijiquan.

After the semester ended, I joined Doctor He's amateur Taijiquan club, which reviewed what we have learned once a month on weekends. In the past 27 years, because of Dr. He's persistent leadership, everyone in the club can firmly remember the Taijiquan they have learned and use it to their benefit.

Dr. He's family has been contributing to the popularization of Taijiquan and the health of the public! Dr. He's husband, Mr. Liu Yaolin, when he was 70 years old, taught us 118 Yang style Taijiquan very carefully on weekends. It took him several months of hard work to transfer the learnings to us. Dr. He's sister, Professor He Murong, came to visit relatives in the United States and was invited to teach us Taiji Ball, Taiji Fan, and the 42 forms of Taiji Sword. Doctor He's son, He Yunsha, also taught us the 55-style Yang-style Taiji sword. In this way, our group of committed students learned many of the 18 styles that have been passed down through Dr. He's family. Before we knew it, we formed a happy community consisting of both Chinese and American practitioners.

Dr. He also often takes us to practice Taijquan in new settings, from mountains to forests to beaches. We go out once a year. From Voyageurs National Park, located on the Canadian side of the U. S. -Canada border to Glacier National Park in Montana to the shore of Lake Superior even to the forests of Brazil and Argentina, there are footprints of our Taijiquan classes everywhere.

In 2010, our happy Taijiquan club went abroad with Dr. He and made took a long voyage through Sichuan, China. In addition to eating wonderful foods and having fun, we also left Taijiquan footprints everywhere. When we were waiting for the flight at Huanglong Airport, we didn't waste the time waiting for the flight. We put our carry-on luggage in order and lined up to practice Taijiquan. At that time, there was a compatriot who came from New Zealand to visit relatives. He introduced himself and said that he also practiced Taijiquan, so he immediately joined the lineup and began to practice with us. Taijiquan also became a way for us to cross barriers, regardless of ethnicity, gender, or nationality.

I am a bit overweight, have small feet, and am often clumsy, so I fall easily. However, since I started practicing Taijiquan, I have not sustained any major injuries after several falls. A few summers ago, I started to walk our family's dog by myself. One day, I tied the leash around my wrist as usual and began our walk. Suddenly, the dog stopped and began chasing a rabbit across the street. By the time I realized what was happening, it was too late! My 105-pound dog yanked me by the wrist so hard I fell. Luckily, right before I hit the ground, my body instinctively utilized the Taijiquan's 2 principles: "The weak will overcome the strong; The soft will overcome the hard." So, while falling, I rolled over. The roll softened the impact, and as I waited for my dog to return to my side, I stood back up and checked to make sure I was ok. Thankfully, I sustained no injuries at all and was completely fine!

Four years ago, I went out for lunch. After walking out of the door, I was focused on talking to my friend and fell quickly without seeing the steps under my feet. In that instant, my body remembered the many hours spent practicing Taijiquan. The soft wins the rigidity and spun around in a rolling way. I got up right away, without any injury or pain.

Last weekend, I went shopping to help boost our state's economy. Back in the parking lot, it was another small step that made me fall. Of course, I rolled very well right away, but unfortunately, I landed on concrete. However, I only sustained minor bruises with no fractures or any type of major injury. After just a few days' rest at home, I was completely fine again!

Thinking back to all these times when I narrowly escaped catastrophe, I feel so grateful and fortunate for my practice of Taijiquan.

The circular motions of Taijiquan make me can turn around and bend down.

Originally, I began practicing Taijiquan to strengthen my body, but somehow, I learned how to save myself in these situations! Each time I finish my practice of Taijiquan, I feel refreshed and happy. My body thanks me each time for the exercise.

For a long time, the quality of my sleep was poor, and I asked the doctor to prescribe medicine. After using it for a week, I didn't want to use it again due to negative side-effects like grogginess and dizziness. I always wanted to use other physical methods. A few months ago, I started practicing Taijiquan in the evening. After practicing Taijiquan, I slept soundly that night, and my sleep index rose. I woke up the next morning and realized that Taijiquan not only is great exercise, but also can be a gentle and relaxing way to improve sleep!

Doing Taijiquan often can enrich and prolong your life. There are so many benefits! In the future, I hope to introduce more people to this art and help everyone overcome the health issues they face.

在学生时代，我常常在文章杂志上读太极拳、气功等等，并不在意。对我而言，那仅仅是中国的文化里的名词。

进入社会工作后，有一阵子，和大多数人一样，迷恋金庸的武侠小说。在"倚天屠龙记"里。武当派掌门人张三丰传授给明教教主张无忌武术。他自己闭关18个月悟出了太极拳、太极剑，打跑了坏人丐帮四大长老之首。太极拳自此深入我的脑海里。

漂洋过海来到美国，也有机缘到中医学院修习中医常识。选修课就必然的选上了太极拳。很幸运，我们由太极拳世家的何新蓉大夫教授太极拳。何大夫很有耐心，循序渐进，手眼身法步一招一招的教我们，教得很仔细，我们也认真地一招一招的学。就这样师生共同努力学会了二十四式太极拳。

学期结束以后，我们加入了何大夫的业余太极拳班。每个月周末复习一次所学，27 年来，因为有何大夫不间断地带领，大伙儿才能牢牢记住所学的太极拳，确确实实的收为己用。

何大夫的先生刘耀麟教授在 70 高龄时很用心地在周末教会了我们 118 式杨式太极拳。花了他好几个月的时间，真是劳苦功高。何大夫的姐姐何慕蓉教授来美国探亲，也被请来传授了我们太极球、太极扇、42 太极剑。何大夫的儿子何云沙也教会了我们 55 式杨式太极剑。如此这般，我们这群好学生一项一项的学，将何大夫家太极武艺学了好多。不知不觉，就形成了一个中西混合的太极班。

何大夫还常常带着我们随时随地练习太极，无论山上、海边。每年我们外出一次。位于美加边境 Voyogeurs 国家公园，蒙大拿州的 Gleciel Park 国家公园，北美最大的淡水湖苏必利湖畔，甚至在巴西、阿根廷，处处都有我们太极班的足迹

2010 年，我们太极班随何大夫出国长征到了中国的四川。除了吃喝玩乐之外，也四处留下太极拳足迹。在黄龙机场候机时，我们没有浪费等机的时间，将随身的行李摆好，便一字的排开，练习太极拳。当时还有一位来之新西兰探亲的同胞，上前自我介绍说他也学过，便马上加入阵容，太极拳打将起来。就这样太极拳不分国籍，不分男女，自然的融合在一起了。

我这个人体重超标了一些，脚又很小，因此很容易跌倒。然而常打太极拳，身体还比较柔软，几次跌倒还没有造成大伤害。几年前一个夏天。我自个去遛狗。为方便健走，特地把狗绳子绑在手腕上。突然，狗儿一停顿，转身瞄准不远的兔子，虽然我马上意识到不妙，但是来不及了，手上的绳子被那个一百零五磅的小子拖到了草地上，摔下我，它就追兔子去了。还好，在人着地之前，我很灵光的想到太极拳的以柔克刚，马上顺势在草地上滚了几滚，减少了正面冲击。坐着等那小子转回来，才站起来摸摸自己，嗯，没事，真幸运啊！

四年前，我外出去午餐。走出门以后只顾说话，没见到脚下的台阶，就很快的往下跌。在那一刹那间，我居然想到不能跌下去，马上就用滚的方式转了一圈，爬起来就这么混过去了，没伤没痛。

上个月的周末，我去逛街买东西，协助促进我们明州的经济。回到停车场，又是一个小台阶，害得我落马。当然啦，马上熟门熟路地打个滚儿，只是滚到了水泥地上，两处肌肉淤青了，还吓了自己一大跳。水泥地可真硬啊，幸好骨头还好好的。后来回家休息三天，也就没事儿了。

回想这几次的"大难不死"也不残，归功于练习太极拳，太极拳的圆形运动让我转得动，弯得下。原本是为了强身健体打太极拳，却意外地救了自己，这可是多出来的收获！今后不光要注意走路，更要持续打太极拳，以期待自己健健康康活到百岁。

我每次练完太极拳，都感到身心舒畅，神清气爽，感到很对得起自己，嗯，今天运动过了。很长一段时间，我睡眠品质很差，找医生开了药，用了一个礼拜以后就不想再用了，因为它有一些副作用，比如头晕、昏昏沉沉的，打算用别的物理方法。前几个月，晚上我们聚会练习太极拳，当晚就睡得很好，睡眠指数上升。我猛然惊醒了：对呀，每次练习太极拳的晚上，一夜好眠。打太极拳温和，动中求静，我怎么早没想到这剂良药呢？

常常打太极拳延年又益寿，好处太多了！在未来，我希望能向更多的人介绍这门艺术，并帮助克服他们所面临的健康问题。

5. Regain My Life 重获新生

By Rose Lo

I love learning, and learning was easy and fun for me when I was young. In second grade, I got accepted to the Art Talent Program in Taipei City, which only admits thirty students per year. After immigrating to the United States, I started taking honors classes in seventh grade, and I took advanced placement classes and college courses during high school. I got good grades every semester and was an honor roll student. I enjoyed solving logical reasoning problems, so I joined the math league and the teacher selected me as one of the team members to represent our school in competitions. I delight in singing and acting; I took concert choir class every semester and participated in school drama performances. I also enjoyed composing poems and making art and some of these writings and paintings have been published and printed in books. I was happy back then, full of dreams and expectations for my future life and work. Unfortunately, before my senior year of high school started, a severe car accident destroyed my aspiration and expectations.

Since then, he has taught Taijiquan voluntarily for 67 years. My mom, who was driving, said that the brakes on our rental car failed, and the car slipped into the ditch in the middle of the highway and rolled onto the lawn not far from the opposite side of the highway. Due to the force of the roll, even though we were wearing seat belts, we were thrown out of the car and fell heavily to the ground. After the accident, I had no idea how long I had been unconscious and only woke up to find that I was no longer inside the car and had blood on my head. I got up and walked towards my unconscious mother, only taking two steps, I felt extreme pain all over my body, and then I fell to the ground with a thud, unable to move. Later, the ambulance took us to the hospital. I had bruises and abrasions all over my body, some bigger than my palm; my back was sore, my head was dizzy, and the doctor sewed several stitches on the cut on my scalp. The cost of hospitalization in the US is expensive, so the doctor saw that I didn't have broken bones and did not find other serious problems, and I was discharged from the hospital the next day.

My school started in less than two weeks, and as a 12th-grade student, I had a busy schedule, and the car accident injuries brought me a lot of difficulties. My whole body was in pain, and my legs were weak, which made walking difficult. I frequently dozed off during class and had trouble concentrating. I hoped to continue getting straight A's through my final year of high school and graduate with the highest honors. Unfortunately, my health was poor, so I only graduated with honors. After I got into college, I thought my health would improve, but it got worse. I used to be full of energy all day, but after the accident no matter how long I rested, my body was still tired. After four hours of class, my body was about to collapse, and I had to sleep for four hours before I could do anything else. I used to have excellent learning ability and memory, but I became forgetful, my brain felt foggy and dizzy, my thinking ability deteriorated, and my language ability declined. I needed to spend twice as much time as others doing homework and studying to get through. My hormones were out of balance, I felt anxious and depressed, my periods became irregular, and my face started to break out with pimples. My back and neck were sore, I had a hard time falling asleep at night and waking up in the morning, I had weak immunity, and I often got sick.

I had two years of chiropractic appointments, massage, and

physical therapy, and I exercised every day, but my condition didn't get better. My family doctor diagnosed me with depression and prescribed antidepressant medication. She said that depression is difficult to cure and that taking medication would get me back to normal. If I do not keep taking the antidepressants, the disease will relapse, therefore I might need to take medication for a lifetime. My former friends alienated me when they learned I was diagnosed with depression. My family felt that my injuries should have fully recovered long ago. Seeing my performance in school getting worse, they were indignant and incredulous, thinking that I had become lazy and deliberately not studying diligently. But studying had become a difficult task for me; since the car accident, I never had sufficient rest, so after one and a half years of college, I quit school temporarily.

My mother felt that my family doctor was not a psychiatry professional and the medication she prescribed was not working for me, so she took me to a psychiatrist. The psychiatrist continued to prescribe me antidepressants. I tried more than a dozen brands of antidepressants, trying each one for at least three months, but none of them worked. I felt increasingly numb, slow to respond, and had panic attacks. My menstrual cycle became severely irregular and during the menstrual period, my whole body was sore, lacked energy, feeling of dizziness, and I was so exhausted I couldn't sit normally in my chair to eat, an indescribable irritable feeling soared to an unbearable level. There were three or four panic attacks every week, and gradually, I had to stop my part-time job, and I couldn't even go to church services and choir practice. My family, relatives, and friends felt that I wasn't working hard and used the car accident as an excuse not to go to school and work. Their constant harsh criticism and mockery made me feel very sad. I couldn't go to school, couldn't work, couldn't speak normally, needed help to go to the toilet, lost self-confidence, and lost all hope and happiness; I felt as though I was dead, bleak, like ashes.

My inner voice told me that I didn't have depression. I had tried more than a dozen antidepressants for years with no improvement; on top of that, my dermatologist prescribed an antibiotic medication for the severe pimples on my face; after taking it for five years, it didn't go away. Therefore, I decided to stop taking all medications.

My mother heard from a colleague that Dr. Xinrong He is an excellent traditional Chinese medicine doctor and suggested I try acupuncture. After four acupuncture sessions, my back pain was relieved, which was more effective than taking painkillers, so I decided to continue with Chinese medicine treatment and participate in the Taijiquan class taught by Dr. He for better health. After doing Taijiquan for half a year, gradually, I no longer needed my parents to drive me to the clinic, and I could go by myself. Not only does Taijiquan make me more energized, it allows my body to repair itself and get a holistic recovery.

Taijiquan is a gentle martial art and I do not feel in danger of getting injured. Practicing Taijiquan is convenient and affordable, and you do not need to buy sports equipment or a specific venue; as long as you exercise gradually and consistently, Taijiquan will improve your entire body and mind. Taijiquan is a moderate-intensity physical activity. After five minutes of exercise, my body warms up, and after twenty minutes, I sweat slightly, and my heart rate and breathing are a little faster. After the practice, I feel my energy flowing smoothly, I am in a good mood, and my whole body is relaxed. I was making progress every day, all symptoms were gradually reducing, and my mind was getting clear. Initially, a car accident ruined my life, but Taijiquan helped me regain my life.

Dr. He cares for her patients with compassion and kindness. She often shared inspirational stories with me and encouraged me not to give up hope and to realize my life dreams. She invited me to work at the clinic to build my confidence and to keep practicing Taijiquan, and we teamed up with friends for a trip to Egypt. An interesting thing happened when we went to Egypt. We heard that camels are very precious in Egypt, each worth a thousand dollars. Since I am single, my friends wanted to find a "Mr. Right" for me. They jokingly asked Egyptian men how many camels they would be willing to offer me as a betrothal gift for marriage. The initial offer was thirty camels, then it increased to a hundred, two hundred; before leaving Egypt, I met a hotel gift shop owner who was willing to marry me with 300 camels and invited me to come to his shop for tea, which was generous. My tour guide said that the word camel is used to address a good-looking girl, and it suits me very well.

Looking back, Dr. He once said that when she first saw me, I looked dull, unresponsive, and felt like a piece of wood, and now, things have changed dramatically. I'm in good health, no longer on medication, in good spirits, beautiful, pursued by people, visiting places, and completed college courses and got a college degree.

I sincerely thank Doctor He, acupuncture, and Taijiquan for bringing me love and miracles.

我喜欢学习，在我年轻的时候，学习对我来说既轻松又有趣。二年级时，考进了全台北市每年只录取三十名学生的美术资优班。移民美国后，我从七年级开始拿了一些荣誉课程，在高中时我拿了先修班和大学课程。我每学期都取得好成绩，是一名荣誉榜学生。我喜欢解逻辑推理问题，所以我加入了数学联赛，老师选择我作为团队成员之一，代表我们学校参加比赛。我喜欢唱歌和表演，每学期都拿合唱班的课，并参加学校戏剧表演。我也喜欢作诗和创作艺术，其中一些作品和绘画被刊登和印刷成书籍。那时的我很幸福，对未来的生活和工作充满了梦想和期待。不幸的是，在我高三开始之前，一场严重的车祸摧毁了我的抱负和期望。

开车的妈妈回忆说，我们租的车刹车失灵，车子滑进了高速公路中间的沟里，滚到了高速公路对面不远处的草坪上。由于翻滚的力量，即使我们系了安全带，我们还是被甩出车外，重重摔倒在地上。事故发生后，我不知道自己昏迷了多久，醒来后发现自己已经不在车内，有许多血从我头上流出。我起身走向昏迷的妈妈，只走了两步，就感到全身剧痛，然后砰的一声倒在地上，动弹不得。后来，救护车把我们送到了医院。我全身都有瘀伤和擦伤，有的比手掌还大；我的背部酸痛，头晕目眩，医生在我头皮的伤口上缝了几针。美国住院费用昂贵，所以医生看我没有骨折，也没有发现其他严重问题，第二天就出院了。

不到两个星期学校就开学了，作为一个 12 年级的学生，我的课业很忙，车祸伤害给我带来了很多困难。我全身疼痛，双腿发软，行走困难。上课时，我常常忍不住打瞌睡，并且注意力无法集中。我希望在高中最后一年持续每科拿 A，以最高荣誉毕业，无奈身体状况很差，我只能荣誉毕业。上大学后，我以为我的健康会有所改善，但却变得越来越严重。以前一整天都精神抖擞，但事故发生后，不管休息多久，身体还是很累。上了四小时课后，我的体力已经不堪重负，我必需要补眠四个小时，才能再做其它事情。我以前学习能力和记忆力都很好，但我变得健忘，脑子有雾，头晕，思维能力下降，语言能力下降。我需要花比其他人多一倍的时间做作业和学习才能勉强完成。我的荷尔蒙失调，我感到焦虑和沮丧，我的月经变得不规律，我的脸上开始长痘痘。我的背部和颈部酸痛，晚上难以入睡，早上起床困难，免疫力低下，经常生病。

我曾经做过两年的整脊、按摩、和物理治疗，我天天锻炼身体，但病情没有任何起色。我的家庭医生诊断我患有忧郁症，开了抗忧郁的药给我。她说忧郁症很难治愈，吃药会帮助我恢复正常的生活。如果我不继续服用抗抑郁药，疾病就会复发，因此我可能需要终生服药。我以前的好友们得知我被诊断出患有抑郁症时就疏远我了。我的家人认为我的伤势早就应该完全康复了，看到我在学校的表现越来越差，他们既愤慨又觉得难以置信，认为我变得懒惰，故意不好好学习。上学对我来说，变得越来越艰辛，自车祸后，我从没得到过充足的休息，于是大学读了一年半后，我暂时休学了。

我妈妈觉得我的家庭医生不是精神科医生，她给我开的药对我没起到效果，于是带我去看精神科医生，精神科医生继续给我开抗抑郁药。我连续试了十几个厂牌的药都没有效用，每个厂牌都尝试了至少三个月，但没有一个有效。我感到越来越麻木，反应迟钝，还引发了恐慌症。经期严重不规律，经期全身酸痛，精神不振，头晕目眩，筋疲力尽，不能正常坐在椅子上吃饭，难以形容的烦躁情绪飙升到我无法忍受的地步。每个星期会有三、四次的惊恐发作，渐渐的，我必须停掉我兼职的工作，我连教会的礼拜和唱诗班练习也无法去了。我的家人、亲戚和朋友都觉得我不够努力，以车祸为借口不去上学和工作。他们不断的冷漠的批评和嘲讽我，使我心里非常难受。我无法上学、无法工作、无法正常说话，连去厕所都需要别人扶我去，失去了自信，失去了所有的希望和快乐，犹如死亡，像灰烬一样卑微而凄凉。

我内心深处的声音告诉我，我并没有忧郁症。这些年来，我尝试了十几种抗忧郁症药，病情从未好转过；除此之外，我脸上的痘痘很严重，皮肤科医生给我开了抗生素药，吃了五年，痘痘也是从未停止长过，因此，我决定停止服用所有药物。我妈妈听同事说何新蓉大夫是位很棒的中医医生，建议我试试针灸。经过四次针灸治疗之后，我的背痛得到了缓解，这比服用止痛药更有效，我决定继续接受中医治疗，并参加何大夫教的太极拳课，锻炼身体。练了半年的太极拳之后，渐渐的，我不再需要爸妈开车送我去诊所，可以自己去了。太极拳不仅让我更加有活力，它使我的身体能够自我修复、得到整体康复。

太极拳是动作柔和的武术，也不重复的做同一个动作，所以我不担心它会导致我运动受伤。用太极拳锻炼身体非常方便实惠，不需要买运动器材，也不需要特定的场地，只要循序渐进、持之以恒的锻炼，整个身心就会获得极大的改善。太极拳动作看似缓慢，其实它是一个中等强度的体能活动，我做了五分钟后身体就暖和起来了，做了二十分钟后，我会轻微流汗，心跳和呼吸会稍为加快。练完后，我觉得能量流动顺畅，心情愉悦，全身都很放松。我每天都在进步，各种症状逐渐减轻，头脑越来越清醒，本来我的人生毁于车祸，太极拳帮助我重获新生。

何大夫对病人非常的有爱心，她常常与我分享励志的故事，鼓励我不要放弃希望，要实现自己的人生梦想。她让我来诊所工作，建立信心，持续打太极拳，我们还和朋友组队一起去埃及玩。去埃及的时候发生一件非常有趣的事情，我们听说骆驼在埃及非常珍贵，每只价值一千美元，大家希望替单身的我找到一位如意郎君，就打趣的到处问埃及的男士们愿意用多少骆驼为聘礼来娶我。一开始是三十只骆驼，然后增加到一百、两百，离开埃及之前，遇到一位酒店礼品店老板，他愿意用三百只娶我，还邀请我到他店里来喝茶，真是豪爽。因此埃及人给我取了一个名字叫小骆驼，我的导游说骆驼是用来称呼漂亮的女生的，很适合我。

回想以前，何大夫曾说，她第一次见到我的时候，我看起来目光呆滞，反应迟钝，感觉就像一块木头；如今发生了翻天复地的变化，我身体情况不错、不再吃药、精神好、漂亮、被人追求、到处去玩，还完成了大学课程、获得大学学位。

我由衷的感谢何大夫、针灸、太极拳带给我爱与奇迹！

6. Taijiquan Relieved My 20 Years of Fibromyalgia
太极拳消除了我 20 年的纤维肌痛

By Sheila Bahl

I first came to see Dr. He on May 23, 2005, for the treatment of chronic back pain and fibromyalgia. I had suffered a whiplash injury in a car accident about 20 years prior to my first visit and had been suffering from chronic headaches, neck pain, and back pain. Eventually, this chronic pain developed into severe fibromyalgia.

I had constant widespread intense muscle pain over much of my body, especially in my back, neck, and shoulders, and also suffered from crushing fatigue and weakness. It was impossible for me to work.

I also suffered from severe pain down my left leg for about two years, I have had a very difficult time walking. I injected cortisone into the lower spine.

I had a very low tolerance for exercise. Any exercise would cause intense pain and spasms in the muscles of my back, especially the upper back and shoulders. I attended a fibromyalgia pool exercise program at the Courage Center for about 4 years, but always had some increase in pain after exercising. Courage sometimes, being in the warm water pool was the only thing that would give me a little respite from the pain and did help my stamina. The pain eventually became too severe to continue even the pool exercise.

I was very weak at the time that I came to see Dr. He. After starting the acupuncture treatments, Dr. He suggested I start taking the Taiji ball class. With my low tolerance to exercise, I thought this would cause pain and severe spasms in my shoulders and upper back. *Taiji* ball is quite aerobic and vigorous and exercises the upper body and arms, but I had no problems with a flare-up in pain, so this helped my endurance and really improved the circulation of *qi* and blood.

After Taiji ball, I studied the 24-form (short form) of *Taijiquan*. It has helped tremendously with my flexibility and strength and helps me prevent back and neck pain. Before I started studying *Taijiquan*, I had a very limited range of motion in my neck and upper back. For many years, whenever I twisted or turned, there was an annoying cracking and grinding sound in my upper back because the ligaments were so tight. Earlier visits to another acupuncturist had alleviated my constant headaches, but I still had much neck and back pain. Over the years, I had many, many physical therapy treatments.

Feldenkreis (note: The Feldenkrais Method is a type of exercise therapy devised by Israeli Moshé Feldenkrais during the mid-20th century. The method is claimed to reorganize connections between the brain and body and so improve body movement and psychological state. Wikipedia) and massage therapy, visits to chiropractors, osteopaths, made it much worse, and neurologist visits (It doesn't work much), trips down to the Mayo clinic for lots of tests including nuclear body scan, EMG, and visits to their fibromyalgia clinic (helped not a bit). So, by the time I came to see Dr. He, I had tried everything with little success

So very gratefully, I now feel an almost entire absence of pain most of the time. The acupuncture, of course, has helped a great deal, but I think that *Taijiquan* has worked to maintain the progress and also strengthen my body enough so that I can function. It has helped my overall energy, endurance, balance, flexibility, and sense of well-being. I notice I can hike on trails that are more difficult and feel freer to exercise or work without worrying about injuring myself or triggering intense pain.

After studying the short form, I have also studied the long form (118), Taiji fan, 42-form Taijiquan, and another form of *Taiji* ball, I have also been able to return to work, which I thought I would never be able to do, and have been working .When I realize the benefits of new things to the body, I like to practice with the group, and I can often talk to myself, reduce my anxiety, let the mood become peaceful, and feel that life is becoming more and more meaningful. I am also getting more and more confident. I also follow Dr. He on a 14-hour plane to China to climb Mount Emei, Huanglong (above 3,000 meters above sea level)

I think Taijiquan remains interesting and challenging, because you can always learn something new no matter how long you have practiced. It is also a great way to reduce stress: slow the mind and instantly bring about. It is also a great way to reduce stress: slow the mind and instantly bring about a sense of calm and peacefulness. I also love it because it is something you can do anywhere and you can do it for your entire life. As I get older, I think it will be a great way to prevent all those aches and pain and stiffness that most people think are a normal part of aging.

Why do I think *Taijiquan* is a good form of exercise for people who suffer from fibromyalgia?

Taijiquan does not have constant repetitive movements. The movements of *Taijiquan* are gentle, varied, and the muscles are moved in many different ways. If a physical therapist or trainer is treating you, the exercises they have you do are very repetitive, often 10 repetitions at a time and maybe multiple sets of these repetitions.

If you have fibromyalgia, your muscles may be extremely tight and have many hard spasms. In my case, any repetitive exercise would cause extreme pain, burning, and even more spasms. Lifting even light weights while doing these exercises would be even worse.

Taijiquan loosens the muscles without stretching. Often, lots of stretching was recommended to treat my hard, spasmed muscles, but this would just cause more pain. Trying to stretch these muscles would make them react by tightening even more; even a massage would sometimes trigger a prolonged flare-up.

The gentle movement of Taijiquan increases qi and blood circulation to the muscles, warms them, and makes them naturally softer and more limber. The muscles loosen as they are moved in many different directions, always moving in gentle circles, not being forced into any position. I can start working again in 20 years. I worked at Dr. He's office for seven years, until I retired

Often people with fibromyalgia lose their stamina and strength because they can't exercise without triggering a bad flare-up of their pain. Taijiquan is strengthening, increases endurance and flexibility, and one is able to practice Taijiquan without causing a flare-up or another type of injury. Therefore, I think Taijiquan is a very beneficial form of exercise for people who suffer from fibromyalgia, and maybe the key to their recovery.

我第一次去看何医生，在 2005 年 5 月 23 日，去治疗我的慢性背痛和纤维肌痛。在来诊所的 20 年前，我在一场车祸中受伤，一直遭受着慢性头痛、颈部疼痛和背部疼痛的折磨。最终，这种慢性疼痛发展成严重的纤维肌痛。

我身体的大部分部位都有持续广泛的剧烈肌肉疼痛，尤其是背部、颈部和肩膀，同时还遭受着极度疲劳和虚弱的折磨。对我来说，工作是不可能的。我的左腿也遭受了严重的疼痛，大约两年，我走路非常困难，脊椎注射了可的松。我对运动的耐受力很低，任何运动都会引起我背部肌肉的剧烈疼痛和痉挛，尤其是上背部和肩膀。我参加了一个 Courage 中心的纤维肌痛症泳池运动项目，大约 4 年，但运动后疼痛总是有所增加，有时在温暖的水池里是唯一能让我从痛苦中得到一点喘息的东西，并帮助了我的耐力。但是疼痛最终变得非常严重，甚至连泳池运动都无法继续。

我去看何医生的时候身体很虚弱。在开始针灸治疗后，何医生建议我开始参加太极球课。由于我对运动的耐受力较低，我认为这会导致肩膀和上背部疼痛和严重痉挛。但太极球课没有让我出现疼痛发作。太极球是一种有氧运动，它能锻炼我的上半身和手臂所以这帮助了我的耐力，并确实改善了气血循环。在太极球之后，我学习了 24 式太极拳。它极大地帮助了我的灵活性和力量，并帮助我防止背部和颈部疼痛。在我开始学习太极拳之前，我的脖子和上背部的活动范围非常有限。多年来，每当我扭动或转身时，我的上背部就会发出恼人的嘎吱声和摩擦声，因为韧带太紧了。早些时候我去看了另一位针灸师，他减轻了我持续不断的头痛，但我的脖子和背部仍然很痛。

多年来，我接受了很多很多物理疗法，Feldenkreis（注：费尔登克雷法是以色列摩西·费尔登克雷法在 20 世纪中期设计的一种运动疗法。该方法被认为可以重组大脑和身体之间的联系，从而改善身体的运动和心理状态。维基百科）和按摩疗法，去看脊椎按摩师，整骨疗法，不太有用，去看神经科医生，吃很多止痛药，去很棒的梅奥诊所做很多测试，包括断层扫描，肌电图。到纤维肌痛诊所就诊，帮助不大。所以，当我去看医生的时候，我已经尝试了所有的方法，但都没有什么成功．

因此，我非常感激太极拳，现在我觉得大部分时间几乎完全没有痛苦。当然，针灸也有很大的帮助，但我认为太极拳有助于保持这个状态，也使我的身体足够强壮，以便我能正常工作。它帮助了我的整体精力、耐力、平衡、灵活性和幸福感。我注意到我可以在更困难的小路上徒步，并且可以更自由地锻炼或工作，而不用担心受伤或引发剧烈的疼痛。

在学了 24 式太极拳之后，我还学习了 42 式及 118 式太极拳，太极扇。后来我还能够重返工作岗位，这在我过去看来是永远也做不到的。当我意识到新事物对身体的好处时，我喜欢和团队一起练习，你可以经常和人交谈，减少焦虑，让情绪变得平静，并感觉生活正在变得越来越有意义！我也越来越自信了。我还跟随何医生乘 14 个小时飞机去中国，爬峨眉山，游黄龙（海拔 3000 米以上）。

我认为太极拳仍然是有趣和具有挑战性的，因为无论你练了多长时间，你总是可以学到新的东西。这也是一个减轻压力的好方法：放慢思维速度，立即带来一种平静和平的感觉。随着年龄的增长，我认为这将是一个很好的方法来防止所有的疼痛和僵硬，而大多数人认为这是衰老的正常部分。

为什么我认为太极拳对纤维肌痛症患者来说是一种很好的锻炼方式？

太极拳没有不断重复的动作。太极拳的动作柔和多样，肌肉以多种不同的方式运动。如果一个物理治疗师或教练在帮助你治疗，他们让你做的练习是非常重复性的，通常一次重复 10.个，可能是多组重复。 如果你患有纤维肌痛症，你的肌肉可能会非常紧绷，有很多严重的痉挛。就我而言，任何重复的锻炼都会导致极度的疼痛、灼烧感，甚至更严重的痉挛。在做这些运动的时候，即使是举重也会更糟糕。

太极拳可以在不拉伸的情况下放松肌肉。通常，医生会建议我做大量的伸展运动来治疗我僵硬、痉挛的肌肉，但这只会引起更多的疼痛。试图拉伸这些肌肉会使它们反应得更紧；即使是按摩有时也会引发长时间的发作。温和的太极拳运动增加了肌肉的气血循环，温暖了肌肉，使肌肉自然地更加柔软和灵活。当肌肉向不同的方向运动时，它们总是以温和的圆圈运动，而不是被强迫到任何位置时，肌肉就会放松。20 年后我又可以开始工作了！我在何医生那里工作了七年，直到我退休。

通常纤维肌痛症患者会失去他们的耐力和力量，因为他们不能在不引发严重疼痛发作的情况下进行锻炼。太极拳加强，增加耐力和灵活性，一个人能够练习太极拳而不引起突发或其它类型的伤害。因此，我认为太极拳对于纤维肌痛症患者来说是一种非常有益的运动方式，可能是他们康复的关键。

　　我非常爱太极拳，可在任何地方练，可以做一辈子。它是克服我肌肉疼痛的最好良药，它是我永远的好朋友！

7. Taijiquan-Best Exercise During Pregnancy 太极拳 - 孕期最佳运动

By Chen Jun

I thought Taijiquan is only for seniors when I was in my twenties. I started to learn Taijiquan because of my best friend, Dr. Xinrong He.

She asked me to be an interpreter for her Taijiquan class in Minnesota. I slowly love this exercise. It is at a slow pace accompanied by deep breathing. It will help people to relax and strengthen the body.

I was so depressed and had trouble sleeping during the period of planning for pregnancy. I can relax after practicing Taijiquan. And I soon got pregnant without fertility treatment. Stay active and involved in the running are kind of hard during pregnancy.

Taijiquan is extremely gentle and a perfect exercise for a pregnant lady.

I had terrible morning sickness in my first trimester. As a pregnant lady, my growing belly makes the center of gravity continuously change. Such body shape changing made me likely to fall over. And in my last trimester, I had horrible lower back pain and hip soreness. I kept practicing 30-60 minutes Taijiquan every day until the day before delivery. Daily Taijiquan exercise helps me to ease my morning sickness and third-trimester discomfort. The slow, deliberate movements practiced in tai chi improve my leg strength and flexibility while also bringing awareness to how to distribute weight across the body. Taijiquan helps my sleeping, balance and increases my stamina which made my labor and delivery easier and quicker.

My baby girl is turning into a teenager now. Everyone loves her since she is a sweet and happy girl. She never gives me hard time. She is an excellent figure skater and has great balance. I think the Tai-chi workout during pregnancy made me stress-free. And it is also a great prenatal education for my baby. My happiness and balance skills got through to the fetus.

Thanks to Dr. He. My family all benefits from Taijiquan. I will keep practicing it for the rest of my life.

以前我一直认为太极拳是老年人锻炼身体的方式，作为一个二十几岁的年轻人自然不屑于学习这个。到了美国明尼苏达，遇到了自己的忘年交朋友 - 何新蓉医生之后，开始接触太极拳。最开始接触太极拳是帮助何医生为太极拳课做翻译。慢慢地就喜欢上了这项运动。太极拳虽然动作看着十分缓慢，但却是一项柔和的有氧运动。还能缓解压力。

我备孕期间精神压力很大，经常失眠，练了太极拳之后心情慢慢放松了下来，没有吃西医的排卵药就自然怀孕有了宝宝。怀孕期间不能从事跑步等大强度的锻炼了。

我发现太极拳是孕期的最佳运动方式。

它是中低等强度的有氧运动，孕妇不用担心剧烈运动造成流产。又可以通过太极拳运动有效地控制体重。太极拳呼吸方式减少怀孕后期气喘的程度。我孕初期严重孕吐，中后期还由于体型体重变化易跌倒，孕晚期更是出现严重的腰痛。我坚持每天 30 分钟到 1 小时的太极拳锻炼直至分娩的前一天，通过这种柔和的锻炼方式，我慢慢发现孕吐好转了，下背痛症状减轻了，同时增强了平衡和免疫力，不容易生病。太极拳帮助我这个孕妇平稳度过整个孕期。

最重要的是太极拳可以使精神得到放松，乐观的情绪也影响到肚子里的宝宝。我女儿现在 15 岁了，是最让家长头疼的青春期孩子，可她依旧性格开朗，学校老师同学都很喜欢她。到哪里都可以交到朋友。另外我女儿从 5 岁开始练习花样滑冰，她平衡感非常好，我认为怀孕期间的太极拳锻炼让我没有压力，这对我的孩子来说也是一个很好的产前教育。我的幸福和平衡技能影响了胎儿，也是受益于我孕期一直练习太极拳。

总之太极拳的好处是数不胜数，我更是感谢何新蓉医生把太极拳推荐给我，让我和家人于生受益。

8. Rehabilitation from Drug Abuse
戒毒后遗症的康复

By Roberto Huerta-Martinez

I, Roberto Huerta-Martinez, had been abusing drugs for 27 years. A major blessing came into my life when I enrolled in the Taijiquan class in May 2010 and began receiving acupuncture under Dr. He's care. Before I decided to be treated with acupuncture, I thought I was going through symptoms of burnout, but I was totally wrong. It was more than burnout. Although my body & soul were in bad shape, my mind didn't want to accept the fact that present times in this declining economy and absorbing as much work as I could be leading me to my grave. I was tired all the time; Monday through Friday, I was looking forward to the weekend, but on Friday afternoons, I was always getting worried and started thinking that the weekend was not enough time to get some rest and was always tired by Sunday afternoon thinking; there I go again; another week at work; the never-ending story; just like the movie (Groundhog Day). I felt that I was dragging myself on my daily routine repeatedly as if every day was the same day. I had the feeling I was not getting anywhere because of the stress that I had voluntarily put on my mind and body simply because I am a responsible person that strives to help people overcome alcohol and drug addiction. I was helping people heal from their addictions, but I was also digging my own grave by working too hard and putting so much stress on my mind and body.

I never considered myself to be a lazy person because I was walking for about half an hour a day on the treadmill and walking a lot in the building I work, but from the moment I began practicing Taijiquan, I noticed that walking is not the exercise the body & mind needs. From the very first acupuncture session after I left Dr. He's office, I felt my energy level increase. My first thought was that as if by a magic touch, Dr. He has made my body & mind feel more relaxed, and I wanted to continue doing things. Before meeting Dr. He, I used to mow the yard and was so tired I had to lay down and take a nap and on the following days I was dragging myself to work, but now, with the help of acupuncture and practicing Taijiquan for at least one hour a day, after mowing the yard, I don't feel like I'm dragging my body anymore. Once again, as if by a magic touch, I feel I can continue doing things around the house. In my childhood, my grandmother taught me that it never hurts anyone to go beyond the call of duty. My grandmother kept me and my brothers and sisters very busy cleaning the house - mopping, sweeping, doing the laundry, etc.; my grandmother could always find something to do. I have always been a busy person and keep myself busy most of the time, but after learning and practicing Taijiquan daily, I now think that Taijiquan is virtually what everybody needs. Taijiquan has helped me reduce my level of stress by about 85% in the past 3 months. Practicing Taijiquan daily works the body & mind and makes you feel like you are creating a miracle for your health and well-being. Today, I don't have to feel embarrassed anymore to openly tell anyone that I was totally burned out because that phase of my life is now over. Before I learned to practice Taijiquan, I had no doubt in my mind that I was merely existing, but today, I feel confident to tell anyone that I'm living a healthier life.

Once I learned the principal steps of Taijiquan, I began practicing Taijiquan once or twice a day to strengthen my body, (especially my knees). I was not used to shifting my body weight in these ways and lacked balance. My first thought was that it would be very difficult to practice this exercise because of all the pain I felt in my body from head to toe, but I thought, let's give Taijiquan a chance to heal my body. I felt that Taijiquan was not a strenuous exercise that I couldn't handle like running or walking at a fast pace. I figured that if I was feeling pain, the pain was associated with the muscles of my body that were not being used, and that is the key element I began to understand from the very first Taijiquan class. I learned from Dr. He that one needs to understand that the slow motion of the movements of Taijiquan is the mechanisms that help massage the internal organs and muscles and help bring the flow of blood to the joints of the body as a source of lubrication. I could move my knees and flex all my joints with a lot more ease as time went by practicing Taijiquan. I know that when starting a new form of exercise, it is easy to immediately have negative thoughts about the new exercise because of the pain that is felt in the body. But it's important to understand that the negative thoughts are only due to the body's inexperience with moving itself in these new ways.

During the first week of the Taijiquan class, I began practicing the first steps as much as I could, but I noticed on the second & third days, I was feeling an unusual pain in my knees and waist and decided to go slower and reduced practicing to about 10 to 15 minutes a day. As time went by, I increased the time practicing gradually, and now, I practice Taijiquan for about an average of 60 to 90 minutes a day. Every morning when I wake up, I warm up my body, then I take a shower, and after the shower, I practice Taijiquan 2 times before eating breakfast, and I practice Taijiquan about 4 times before lunchtime. Before and after supper, I practice Taijiquan about 5 more times. Late in the afternoon, I spend about 1 hour meditating. I don't watch T.V. or do anything else before bed - I just go to my bedroom, lay in bed, close my eyes, and imagine

I'm in *paradise*. I stretch my whole body, flexing my arms and rotating my shoulders and my legs while I'm lying in my bed. What I mean about paradise is to place my mind away from work and try to relax and release stress from my brain caused by the hard work of my daily routine.

Every now and then I remember that when I was in college, one of my teachers used to say, "it never hurts to exercise the brain", but the work I do counseling clients requires that I do critical decisions, and I feel as if "I'm lifting" about 200 cases at any given time helping others overcome alcohol and drug addiction. I'm not complaining because I love the work I do; I have been about 17 years sober and understanding the seriousness of alcohol and drug addiction is what drives me to continue working hard to help others survive another day. Today, I have no doubt in my mind that the day I began learning Taijiquan under Dr. Xin Rong He's supervision, my mind & body has developed the skill one needs to live a happier and healthier life. Today I'm able to concentrate better and think more clearly, and I don't feel as much stress as I did before I met Dr. He. Throughout the care of acupuncture & Taijiquan training, my memory & concentration is 100% better. I'm no longer feeling the pain I once felt in my body after mowing the yard because Taijiquan has eliminated what I call, the side effects of doing hard labor. I was also wrong to think that mowing the yard & raking the leaves was hard work. I was wrong to think this way because I am almost 55 years old and before I met Dr. He, I had concluded that all the mental, physical, and emotional pain and stress were associated to getting older. Today I don't think this way; there's no such thing as accepting pain and agony due to aging because today, by simply practicing Taijiquan, my life has taken a 180-degree turn. I wake up in the morning and look forward to practicing Taijiquan throughout the day. Before I go to sleep, I think about how fortunate I am to have met Dr. He because Dr. He is really a person that helps people heal from the inside out. I have no doubt in my mind that her patients feel 100% better from the moment they walk out the door after the first visit and look forward to coming back again and again. Mentally, physically, and emotionally, my life has made a turn in a positive direction because of Dr. He's help.

I started to observe my body during Taijiquan practice. Initially, I felt some pain when I flexed my knees and rotated my waist from left to right. However, I quickly realized that the key component to addressing this pain was to practice these gentle movements as many times as possible throughout the day and that my body would get used to these motions. Eventually, the pain subsided, and I was able to gain greater control over my whole body when practicing Taijiquan. I do believe that no matter your age or physical condition, you can start doing at least basic movements in certain parts of the body to feel better and alleviate pain.

People recovering from alcohol, drug, and tobacco addiction often develop chronic pain due to a lack of physical activity. Taijiquan, without a doubt in my mind, is another key component to bettering their lives and dealing with chronic pain. Taijiquan brought immediate results to my mind and especially my body.

People with lower back pain get positive results practicing Taijiquan daily. I got a lower back injury when I was about 17 years old. I fell from a roof 2 times because I was working as a laborer in roofing. I was very young then, and I fell about 12 to 15 feet twice, both landing on my back, but because I was young, I didn't feel I was injured; I just fell, bounced, and went back to the roof worried I was going to get fired for falling off the roof.

Anyways, the pain in my lower back did manifest when I was in my 30s. I was no longer able to work in construction and was no longer able to lift more than 80 or 100 lbs. I have been wearing a back brace, very tight to my stomach because of the back pain, but ever since I have

42

been practicing Taijiquan, once again, as if by a magic touch, the pain in my lower back has almost disappeared. I get tired working, walking for about one hour a day, but after practicing Taijiquan throughout the day the feeling of fatigue is no longer there.

I also suffered from Carpal Tunnel for about 5 years, but in the last 3 months, Taijiquan has helped me relieve the constant pain and burning feeling I used to feel. The gentle Taijiquan movements have helped me feel better, and now when I rotate my wrists, hands, and shoulders, I no longer feel the pain and burning I once felt. Taijiquan has relieved all the pain I used to have. Today I feel a whole lot better thanks to Dr. He.

I'm so excited about the remarkable changes to my mind & body that I have experienced. I recommend Dr. He's Taijiquan class and acupuncture to all my coworkers, clients, friends, and family members.

I, Roberto Huerta-Martinez, feel honored to give permission to Dr. He to use my descriptions in full or in part for her book. Dr. He is so remarkably humble, yet, very respectful in providing her professional work to all her patients. Thank you so very much, Dr. He. I will be your patient for as long as I live, and I really consider you to be the master of healing peoples' lives.

我是罗伯托·许尔塔-马丁内兹,有 27 年的吸毒史。受主的祝福,在 2010 年 5 月学习了太极拳及接受何大夫的针灸治疗。在决定针灸以前,我的身体和灵魂都极糟,我的心已接受不了低落的经济及超负荷的工作,我感到自己快钻到坟墓里去了。从周一到星期五我都很累,我盼望周末到来,我需要休息。星期天下午我又会想明天又要工作了,工作真做不完,就象电影"偷天情缘"(Groundhog Day 土拨鼠节),表示每天重复一样的工作。就像每天都是同样的,我觉得我身体不会好了。因我是一个负责任的人,我的工作是帮助许多人戒毒戒瘾,我从来不是一个懒人,我每天要走一个半小时去工作的地方,在那儿还要走很多路,我累的筋疲力竭。

从第一次做针灸起，我就很有精神了。我第一感觉就像变魔术那样，让我放松了。而当我练太极拳后，走路就不算啥了。在我遇到何大夫之前，我在家要剪草，累得要躺下打盹，第二天还要拖着腿去上班。但现在好多了，在太极拳帮助下，剪草后不太累。就像被神力触碰一样，在家中可做更多的事情。我从小从奶奶那里学到的就是多干活，找事做，洗衣擦地等。所以我习惯将自己变成忙碌的人。

我的一生都忙都累。但是学了太极拳后，帮我恢复了健康与平静。在过去的 3 个月，我减低了 85% 的劳累。天天练，天天有奇迹发生。

练太极拳前，我累得快死过去了，快不存在了。但是今天我可自信地告诉大家，我现在过的是健康的生活，劳累从我生命中消失了。

我第一次练太极拳时，认为太难，从头到脚都酸痛，因为我的膝盖很不好，总是平衡不了重心。但我还是想试试。

现在我觉得太极拳并不难，它不象走、跑那样快，酸痛是因为有部份肌肉关节过去未用到过，这是很重要的一点。自己要明白，不要有负面想法。

何大夫教我们太极拳做慢动作是一个很重要的方法，可按摩肌肉及内脏，增加血液循环，产生胶质样东西帮助关节灵活。所以第一周练太极拳时，第二三天膝盖手腕特酸痛，所以一天只练 2 分钟。以后我每天在早饭前练，下午吃饭前还练。晚上，我也不看电视，躺在房间里冥想，想象在天堂里还做伸展运动。我所说的天堂是在我脑海中没有工作，没劳累，不烦恼，总之一切都放松。

想起我上大学时，一个老师曾经说过，多动脑子好。我现在是背负着帮助 200 个吸毒者的责任，我从不抱怨，因我喜欢我的工作。我已 17 年不用毒品了，我知道喝酒吸毒的严重后果，我要努力帮助他们活下来。让他们戒毒戒酒。

毫无疑问，当我开始上何大夫的课时，我的身心就开始健康快乐起来，我的注意力更集中，思想也更清楚，也没有以前那样劳累了。经由针灸和太极拳的帮助，我的记忆和注意力都上升了 100%。在我剪草后，身体也不再感到疼痛了，因为太极拳帮我消除了劳动过多症（我自称）。

练太极拳时，我开始注意练我的姿势，以腰为轴，站稳脚步，在做云手时运用手栏般地看过去。刚开始练太极拳时，我发觉伸展膝关节和转腰时会疼痛，但我明白每天练习这些动作是重要的关键。身体会渐渐习惯这些动作，有利于帮助全身放松。我相信那些有疼痛练太极拳的人们，不论是年纪大了，或是其他的原因，至少可以由练膝盖和转腰动作来帮助止痛。

人们在用酒、毒品过久，通常会发展成慢性疼痛。原因是运动不够。但毫无疑问的太极拳是帮助慢性疼痛的另一关键，太极拳在短时间之内就给了我立竿见影的好效果，帮助我的心、身健康起来了。

当我17岁时我的腰部受伤，我从屋顶上跌下来两次，因为我是做屋顶的工人，跌下来时，我背着地，因为那时年轻，并不觉得受了伤，下跌还反弹一下。30岁后我才明显感到背痛。我不能在工地做事了，也不能再提重东西，我一直带着腰带，紧紧的束起肚子。但是自从我开始练太极拳后，就觉得象是被施了神法一样，我的腰痛烟消云散了，工作累了练练太极拳，那精疲力尽的感觉就不再存在。太极拳使我之前所有的疼痛减轻到最低程度。我患手腕疼痛5年，但在过去3个月通过旋转练习，我的手腕和肩膀彻底消除了火烧感。

在没有遇到何大夫之前，我对自己下了个定论，就是我所有的智、身、心劳累与疼痛来自於我的老化。现在我不这样想了，我错了，老化就得疼痛的活着吗？我才55岁，不老。练太极拳使我的生命180度的大转变，从早上醒来到睡觉前，我都期盼着练太极拳。我想着自己有多幸运，可以遇见何大夫，因为她真心的关心病人，从内到外的医治人，我相信病人在走进她的诊所后就100%舒畅起来，而且希望再次回来。我的智、身、心已有重大的改变，谢谢何大夫，我和妻子会有着更健康快乐的生活．

我为我身心的变化觉得非常兴奋，我建议我同事、客户、朋友及家人向何大夫学太极拳和做针灸，非常谢谢您，何大夫！我想一辈子做你的病人．

9. Slimming Secret 苗条秘方

By Joan Saum LADC

Beginning in 2004, I learned Taijiquan from Dr. He. Taijiquan brought many benefits for me. It greatly improved the quality of my sleep, improved my digestion, and my mood became more and more happy, even in everyday life. Others even said I became healthier and more beautiful!

For the first time in my life, I did not need to fight for my body weight. Back in high school, my height was 5.5 feet and I weighed 115 pounds - I felt fat and started to lose weight. I tried all the methods but still gained weight; I ended up weighing 185 pounds by age 25. I battled for the next 20 years, losing and gaining weight in a terrible cycle, and ended up becoming a girl who was addicted to losing weight. I starved myself and became a monster, but I just could not lose the weight for good.

I would like to become leaner, but as soon as I stop those crazy weight loss methods, the weight always came back. Since I began practicing Taijiquan, I gradually reduced my weight and my weight stabilized; I realized that Taijiquan completely changed my life!

I now weigh 145 pounds; I can safely eat what I want to eat. I don't have any more food quirks or feel extreme hunger anymore. I am no longer addicted to sweet and greasy foods. When I want to eat, I can manage to eat only eat a small amount of food, so I now can enjoy eating, and no longer have guilt and panic disorder. I also no longer worry about gaining weight.

Many sources preach heavy exercise that produces sweat and fatigue as the solution to fat loss; I'm here to tell you that you really can lose weight by practicing Taijiquan. Taijiquan was the answer to my weight loss!

Taijiquan is a treasure.Taijiquan is a slimming Secret.

我从 2004 年开始向何大夫学习太极拳，我现在非常享受太极拳给我带来的许多好处。睡眠质量大大改善，消化功能提高了，心情变得越来越愉快，每天都高高兴兴的生活。别人都说我变的更健康漂亮了！

我生命中开始第一次不需要与体重作斗争，早在中学时代，我的身高 5.5 尺，体重 115 磅，我觉得自己很胖，开始减肥，我试了所有的方法，体重还是上升，到 25 岁时已达 185 磅了，与体重搏斗了 20 年，但我减了又增，增了又减，变成减肥上瘾的女孩子，我把自己饿坏了，我简直成了一个减肥的怪兽，但是却总是不能减低体重。

我拟减一些肥，但只要停止疯狂减肥方法，体重马上会回来。自从练了太极拳以后，我的体重逐渐减低并开始稳定了，我也意识到太极拳使我的生命完全地改变了！

我现在体重 145 磅，我可以安心地要吃我要吃的东西。再无食物怪癖，我不再感到肚子饿，我也不再对甜、油腻食物上瘾，如果想吃的时候，我可以有控制的只吃少量食物，故现在可享受吃东西了，不再有罪恶感和惊恐症了。也不再担心体重会增加了，许多减肥的方法要有流汗与劳累才能减，那不是真的！真的是练太极拳就能减肥。太极拳是减肥的答案！

太极拳是个宝，太极拳是苗条秘方。

10. Taijiquan Became my Version of Coffee
太极拳是我离不开的咖啡

By Andy Reichert

I began learning the short-form of Taijiquan more than two years ago, and soon after I became a patient at Dr. He's acupuncture clinic in a search for better overall health. I had spent the previous five winters fighting long, drawn-out colds and never feeling completely rested. Even in the summer I frequently felt lethargic and drained, a very frustrating experience on beautiful, warm, and sunny days.

When Dr.He told me about the upcoming *Taijiquan* class and how it could help keep my immune system become balanced and strong, I knew I needed to follow through with it. I had a brief exposure to *Taijiquan* ten years earlier and wanted to practice it then but could not find a way to make it fit into my schedule.

As a college student and competitive cyclist, my days were pretty well filled up, especially weekends spent racing.

Taijiquan class started in early January, and I showed up the first day feeling better than I had in a while. The acupuncture was definitely helping and I was excited to be healthy and full of energy at a time of year when I had often been sick and drained of energy. I knew about halfway through the first class that *Taijiquan* was physically more difficult than it looked (in part because of repeated practice and long holds), but I was able to pick up the forms relatively quickly. I diligently practiced five days a week for at least 30 minutes and then went to our 3-hour class every Saturday afternoon.

Even from the beginning, I could tell that *Taijiquan* was having a positive effect on my body. My chronically tight neck and shoulders began to loosen, my balance became more confident, and my ability to hold a form or pose for a long time grew. When the first bike rides of late-winter/earlier-spring began, I could tell something was different. In the previous 15 years of early season rides, I traditionally struggled to keep pedaling strongly for the first few weekends of three-hour rides and often came home with a sore and stiff neck and aching shoulders. This time though, I finished my first three-hour ride with just as much energy as I had when I began and there was no pain in my neck or shoulders. My legs felt stronger and had more "snap" on the hills, and I was ready to ride again the next day, free of any soreness.

It wasn't until we learned the last form, though, that I felt a complete sense of balance, mentally, and physically. I literally felt like my brain had grown new synapses and connections over the previous three months and practicing the complete short form from *Taijiquan* left me with a slight buzzing feeling throughout my body. Because I often seek out new challenges, I decided that once I had the complete short form down, I would add a new twist: in addition to starting to the left (as we learned from Dr. He), I would teach myself how to do the complete short from starting to the right. Although this seems logically easy, it presents a much more demanding challenge physically and mentally. I soon realized that "reversing" all 24 forms required an intense amount of focus and determination, let alone balance and strength. After a few weeks of practicing starting to the right, I had the general flow of movements down and was on making it look and feel as smooth as starting to the left.

Soon after I was able to start to either side with equal skill, around mid-May, I moved my *Taijiquan* practice from the afternoon/evening to first thing in the morning. Although it was tough to give up thirty minutes of quiet reading time before breakfast, waking with *Taijiquan* was wonderful. Even on the toughest morning, I felt invigorated and ready to start my day.

Taijiquan became my version of coffee – I wasn't exactly surly without it, but I was more alert and cheerful when I started my day with *Taijiquan*. I found that *Taijiquan* first thing was a great way to warm up my body for an early bike ride or a run.

By the time June came, I had made it through an entire cold season without a cold. I know that acupuncture helped me get my energy back and restore my immune system, but *Taijiquan* helped me maintain both. That summer, I never had one day where I felt like I was dragging. I had some very stressful days at work, but I always made time for *Taijiquan*, even if it was later in the day. By the end of summer, I was starting to try *Taijiquan* with my eyes closed (try balancing on one leg with your eyes closed, then imagine the challenges of moving through *Taijiquan* forms while keeping them closed). After a while, I was able to make it through without tipping over or grabbing on to something to stay upright.

Since that summer, I have continued to practice *Taijiquan* four to six times a week. When the weather is above 40 and not pouring rain, I am in my backyard, enjoying the bird songs as the day wakes. When it's colder or too wet, I move to my basement. I can't say that I haven't been sick at all in the last two years, but I can say that colds come much less frequently than they did. Even when I do get sick, I still practice every morning to get some relief from the symptoms and speed up the recovery. I still feel good after long early-season bike rides, even when they approach four hours in late February. I'm still a little amazed that I come home without stiff and sore muscles; I certainly still get tired, but it's a good, relaxing state of being tired, not an uncomfortable and stiff zombie-like state that I used to know so well.

My most recent challenge is to slow my practice down, way down. A friend in Seattle told me about his *Taijiquan* instructor, who said that a complete short form should take six minutes. I don't always have enough time each morning to do this, but I do try to work on fluidity and slowness at least once or twice a week. I've found that it's really difficult to slow it down enough to fill six minutes, but I've been getting closer with more consistent practice. I do know that *Taijiquan* will continue to be a life-long practice and that I will keep finding new ways to challenge myself with. Next up – learning the long-form of *Taijiquan* as soon as I can fit the time in again.

为了我的全身的健康，我成为何大夫针灸诊所的病人。两年多前，我开始练二十四式太极拳。过去的5个冬天我的感冒一直不好，也得不着很好的休息。即使在夏天，我也常昏睡无力，在美好、温暖、充满阳光的日子感到无奈。当何大夫告诉我上太极拳课能帮助提升和强化我的免疫力，我知道这是我需要做的事。十年前我接触太极拳时很想练，但挤不出时间。我上大学时是一个越野赛车手，我每天很忙，而且周末要比赛。

太极拳课在一月开始。第一天我感到非常好，针灸也的确帮助了我许多，我很高兴。现在健康了有力气，我在学太极拳课时我就知道了看着容易做起来难，而且有许多姿势要长时间保持，但我很高兴很快地学这些姿势，我认真地练，每周5天，每次30分钟，每周上3小时课。

从开始学太极拳，就对我身体有很好的影响，紧绷的颈部开始放松，对平衡有助，我能够较持久做动作，所以我在去年冬天到早春的骑车运动，我感到有所不同了。过去的15年每个早春骑车运动，我一般要化很多力气踩踏板，在前几周3小时骑车会脖子肩背痛，但现在已较好了。我不仅完成3小时训练，还很有精神，肩颈未痛，我的腿更强壮更有韧性了，在隔天的山上骑车时，我没有任何地方疼痛。

当学太极拳最后一个动作时，我感到精神身体都平衡了。我觉得有新的道路了。在过去 3 个月在练习 24 式太极拳时，身体感到气在流动，我感到新的挑战，我决定了学会 24 式之后，还要学新的东西，太极拳除了从左边抱球，还要从右边抱球，虽然看起来很简单，但对我有许多挑战，尤其是拗步，需很多注意力和决心、平衡和力量，在几周练习太极拳后，我开始觉得很顺了。

很快我两边练都顺了，5 月中旬时，我把太极拳的中晚上练习挪到早上，要这 30 分钟读书时间用掉很难，但为了与太极拳一起醒来那是很美好的事，甚至在最糟的早晨，我也准备好了一天的挑战去练太极拳。

太极拳是我离不开的咖啡！太极拳帮助我非常清醒快乐。

我还觉得太极拳是一个很好的暖身运动。到六月来的时候，我已经度过了一整个寒冷的季节，在寒冷的季节我没生过一次病。我知道针灸帮助我恢复能量，提升免疫力，但太极拳帮助维持保住它，我都很喜欢。在炎热夏天，我没有像吸毒人那样一昏一沉的感觉。一天工作下来我很劳累，但一定保留时间复习太极拳，即是太晚，我也练太极拳。

夏天之后我闭着眼练太极拳，用一只腿站着一会后就不需要抓东西保持平衡了，自从夏天后我会连续练 4—6 次。当气温 40 度没下雨时我在后院欣赏鸟儿唱歌，如天气太冷太湿我会去楼下。我不敢说这两年没生过病，但感冒少多了。甚至生病了还要练太极拳，好帮助我恢复。我喜欢早春骑车，一直到二月底我接近骑 4 小时。我仍然有点惊讶的是，我回到家的肌肉没有僵硬和酸痛，我当然仍然很累，但这是一种良好的、放松的疲劳状态，而不是我以前很熟悉的不舒服的、类似僵尸的僵硬的状态。

我最近的挑战是把太极拳动作放得很慢。我的朋友在西雅图的太极拳老师讲要 6 分钟做完 24 式，我平常晨起没有时间，但我会找个时间慢慢完成，每周做 1-2 次，我发觉放慢动作 6 分钟很难，但已接近了。我知道我会一辈子练太极拳。

下一个挑战是学长的太极拳

推荐太极拳给任何想要提升免疫力，增强体力和减轻压力的人们。

11. Improved my Intelligence Level
开发智力

By Huang Heyu

In 1989, I was lucky to have the chance to know Mr. He Ming and started to learn *Taijiquan* from him. At that time, I did not anticipate how my life was going to benefit from it, but I did not have to wait long to see what happened two years later.

Before I started practicing *Taijiquan*, I was known as the one who caught a cold as often as the weather changed. For others, to recover from the cold takes only one week; for me, it could be as long as two weeks or sometimes even a month. However, everything changed after I started practicing *Taijiquan*. I was surprised to find that my immune system seemed to improve a lot, since I turned out to be the only person in my family who stay untouched and healthy even when the severest flu was going around. When my family fell ill, three of my four people were bedridden with high fever, but I had no problem. Meanwhile, people all say that I have a better complexion with healthy hues all the time.

For the last two decades, a large part of my work is writing. Unfortunately, the neck disease I had caused many problems such as dizziness and memory-loss that had largely affected my working efficiency. However, all these symptoms disappeared gradually once I started to practice *Taijiquan*.

The 2000 year, I published around 166 reports and articles, 8 academic papers on management, and one book, which was more publications than in 1988 and 1989 combined! I cannot imagine all these could be achieved if not because of *Taijiquan*, which has cleared my mind and improved my memory and energy level. I have never felt better and been more efficient in my life. All my works have kept on receiving very positive reviews. Once I even finished writing a 1600-word article within 80 minutes! With an improved intelligence level, I am capable of doing many things that I was not before.

Before, the dizziness had limited my daily activities and I seldom went out even to the suburbs of Beijing. During the six years between 1983 and 1988, I only traveled once.

However, when *Taijiquan* became part of my life, I no longer had such problems anymore, and just in 2000 year，I made six domestic and one international trip. Although the flight to West Germany was more than 10 hours, I did not find it unbearable at all.

I achieved this result by relying on Mr. He Ming's guidance and by my own persistence in practicing Taijiquan, namely "Sanfu (the three most hot periods)" in summer and "Sanjiu (nine coldest periods)" in winter.

1989 年，我很幸运地有机会认识了何明先生，并从他那里开始学习太极拳。当时，我并没有预料到我的生活将如何从中受益，但我没有等多久就能看到两年后发生了什么。在我开始练习太极拳之前，我是一个因天气变化而经常感冒的人。对其他人来说，从寒冷中恢复只需要一个星期；对我来说，这个时间可能长达两周，有时甚至是一个月。然而，在我开始练习太极拳后，一切都变了。我惊讶地发现，我的免疫系统似乎有了很大的改善，因为我是家里唯一的一个即使是最严重的流感也能保持健康的人。当家人生病时，我家四个人中有三个人因高烧卧床不起，但我没有问题。与此同时，人们都说我的肤色一直很健康。

在过去的二十年里，我的大部分工作都是写作。不幸的是，我的颈部疾病引起了很多问题，比如头晕和记忆力减退，这在很大程度上影响了我的工作效率。然而，当我开始练习太极拳时，所有这些症状都逐渐消失了。

2000 年，我发表了大约 166 篇报告和文章，8 篇关于管理的学术论文和一本书，比 1988 年和 1989 年的总和还要多！如果不是因为太极拳，我无法想象所有这些都已经使我的头脑清醒，提高了我的记忆和精力水平。在我的生活中，我从来没有这样感觉好，更有效率。我所有的作品都得到了非常积极的评价。有一次，我甚至在80 分钟内写完了一篇 1600 字的文章！随着智力水平的提高，我能够做很多我以前没能做的事情。

以前，头晕限制了我的日常活动，我很少去北京的郊区。在1983 年到 1988 年的六年里，我只旅行过一次。

然而，当太极拳成为我生活的一部分时，我就不再有这样的问题了，在 2000 年，我做了六次国内旅行和一次国际旅行。虽然飞往西德的航班超过 10 个小时，但我并不觉得无法忍受。

我取得这样的结果，是依靠何明先生的指导，以及依靠自己的坚持练太极拳，即夏练"三伏"和冬练"三九"。

12. Taijiquan Gives Me the Courage
太极拳给我勇气

By Dr. Xinrong He

About 20 years ago, I attended the graduation ceremony of my friend's daughter in the UK. One day I went to Scotland with my friends, and we took the train home in the evening, but the train was late and arrived at the destination very late. From the train station to the accommodation, we had to pass through a small alley. I saw three young people standing at the entrance of the alley, asking for money from passersby. But our money was all gone, and the remaining money was placed at a friend's house. At that time, the sky was overcast with drizzle, the cold wind was biting, and the streetlights flickered like a ghost fire, which made people feel depressed and scared. What were we to do?

At this time, the image of my fearless father came to my mind: once on the bus, a few thieves stole money from a farmer. My father found out and asked them to hand over the money. When the thieves saw that my father was a skinny old man, they rushed at my father and threatened him to stay out of their way. My father used Taijiquan's "White Crane Spreads Its Wings" to throw a thief over a long distance; to the other who tried to hit my father with his fist, my father used Taijiquan's "Grasp the Bird's Tail" to throw the man to the ground. Seeing that, those thieves said, "bad luck, we met a master", so they had to give the money back to the farmer obediently.

Thinking of my father's bravery, I immediately said to my friends with enthusiasm: "I practiced Taijiquan with my father since I was a child. If they want to attack us because we have no money, we will fight back with Taijiquan. I will hit the skinny guy on the temples with Taijiquan's "Strike Opponent's Ears with Both Fists" and "white crane spreads its wings"made he see stars and don't know where to go, and you punch other guys in their nose and let them wipe their noses, then we run …" So, my friends and I walked forward strutting and singing, and amazingly they just stared, oh, overwhelmed by our heroism! We crossed the alley safely. However, I am a little regretful. I am 74 years old this year, and I no longer have a chance to fight again. I should have used Taijiquan to teach those bad boys a lesson!

Later, when I was going back to America, my friend, his daughter and I took the subway to the airport. We were about to get on the subway, and suddenly I saw an advertisement for the third episode of Harry Potter. I liked this movie very much and stopped to watch the advertisement. When I come back to my senses, my friend was already on the subway, which was about to leave! My friends were desperately calling me to get on the subway, as I otherwise would have been left behind, lost. As the subway door was closing, I immediately sprinted, and used Taijiquan's "Kick with Right Heel" to hold the subway door, and got my head and body in. I heard a "pop", the door was completely closed, and my backpack was stuck in outside the subway door. As people on the subway extended their thumbs to praise me as a warrior, I secretly prayed that the camera and video recorder in my backpack would not be damaged. That is a precious souvenir of traveling to the UK!

It was Taijiquan that gave me courage and strength! I hope to complete another trip to the UK smoothly and happily!

大约是 20 年前，我去英国参加友人女儿的毕业典礼。有一天与友人去苏格兰玩，傍晚乘火车回家，可是火车误点了，很晚才达目的地。而从火车站到住宿处要经过一个小巷道，只见巷口有 3 个年轻人站在那里，凡是过路之人他们都伸手要钱。可是我们的钱化光了，余钱放在友人的女儿家，当时天阴沉沉的，下着毛毛雨，冷风刺骨，路灯暗暗的闪一闪的像鬼火，让人心情很压抑。怎么办？这时父亲路见不平，拔刀相助的大无畏形象在我脑海浮出：一次在公交车里有几个小偷偷了一个农民的钱，被我父亲发现了，父亲让将钱交出来。他们一看是个干巴老头，便扑向我父亲，还骂少管闲事。父亲用太极拳的"白鹤亮翅"，将其中一人靠过去老远；对另一个挥着拳头打来的人，父亲用太极拳的"揽雀尾"的履法将那人摔到地上，那几人一看连连说"倒霉，遇到高手了"，只好乖乖地还钱了……。顿时我热血沸腾地对朋友讲："我从小随父亲练太极拳，如果没钱要打架的话，我们就用太极拳回击。我用"双峰贯耳"打那个瘦子的太阳穴，让他眼冒金花不知所措，另外一人你用拳头打他的鼻子，让鼻子酸溜溜擦鼻涕时，咱们就跑……。"于是我和朋友雄起起气昂昂地挺胸阔步唱着歌向前走，令人惊讶的是他们只呆呆地看着，哦，被我们的英雄气概压下去了！我们平安的过巷口了。不过，我倒是有点遗憾，今年 74 岁，再没有机会打架了，就该用太极拳教训教训那坏小子！

后来我要回美国了，友人与女儿送我。我们三人准备上地铁，忽然我看到广告，哈利波特第三集即将上演，我很喜欢这个电影，我立即停下看宣传片，等回过神，朋友已经上地铁了，她们拼命地喊我，我疾步跑去，必须上地铁，不然我在哪下车，机场在哪？我是茫茫然。这时地铁门正在徐徐关上，我立即用太极拳"右蹬脚"将车门顶住，头与身体钻进了进去，只听啪一声，车门完全关了，我的背包卡在了车门外。我，立正为大家站岗了，车上的人还伸出大拇指赞我是勇敢的卫士！殊不知我在暗暗祷告，千万不要把背包里的照相机和录像机夹坏了，那可是游英国的珍贵纪念呢！

是太极拳给了我勇气和力量！让我顺利、开心的完成了英国之旅！

13. Finally Find a Job 终于找到工作

By Jin Ming Luo

One month after I was born, I suffered from pneumonia, convulsion, and coma. Although I survived after being rescued by Chongqing Children's Hospital, I was left with sequelae and my body was very weak. When I was 7 years old, my health was even worse, accompanied by a decline in intelligence, dull eyes, twisted mouth for no reason, long-term insomnia and chorea. I struggled to study and didn't even graduate from elementary school. At the age of 13, my hands started to cramp, and at the age of 15, my head began to swing involuntarily from side to side. After 3 years of acupuncture, Chinese herb medicine and massage therapy, my condition had not improved.

At the age of 18, one day my mom told me that some young men living upstairs went to practice Taijiquan every day in a community park. They looked very healthy, and she suggested that I could go with them. That was when Taijiquan entered my life. The earlier days of learning *Taijiquan* were not easy at all. Due to my poor memory and health, nobody believed that I could actually learn it. So, the teacher asked me to stay in the back and follow the rest of the people. While everybody else learned the 24-Form in a week, I needed two months. But I did not feel frustrated or give up; rather, I started to learn the 36-Form within a year, and then the 118-Form and finally, *Taiji* broad sword.

Before, because I always got sick and my speech was so unclear, no company would hire me. However, after one year of practicing *Taijiquan*

60

my health improved greatly. Also improved were my mental abilities, my reactions, and my analytical abilities. After I could communicate with people freely, I was hired by a factory as a laborer. When I received a salary for the first time in my life, I was choked up with happiness. I ran to the park and cried out to my teacher and the other *Taijiquan* practitioners that I had just earned the first paycheck of my life! Everybody was happy for me.

Up to today, I have been practicing *Taijiquan* for 8 years. My hands no longer shake, neither do my mouth or head. Now I have no problem in expressing myself and can communicate easily with others. I am not suffering from insomnia anymore and I can always sleep through the night. I also learned the *Taiji* push-hands, and I have always been the winner when playing with others.

After practicing *Taijiquan* for the last 8 years, my health has been improving a lot; however, my speaking ability is still not as good as other people's. Therefore, I need to keep on doing *Taijiquan*.

Taijiquan let me have a second chance at life. Now I can work and support myself. If not for *Taijiquan*, I think I would have to depend on others for the rest of my life.

Taijiquan,—Let me finally find a job！

我出生后一个月就患肺炎，抽风，昏迷。经重庆市儿童医院抢救才活过来。但留下后遗症，身体也很虚弱。到 7 岁时身体更差，智力日减，双眼呆滞，嘴巴无故扭动，长期失眠，并有舞蹈病等现象，读书费力，小学都未能毕业。13 岁时双手开始痉挛。15 岁那年，头又开始不由自主地左右摆个不停。扎针，服中药，推拿 3 年均未见效。

18 岁时，有一次妈妈对我说："楼上住的几位年轻人天天练拳，身体都很好，你也去练练吧"！于是我到沙坪公园武术站学习太极拳。我的记忆力差，手脚又不灵，加上那副病相，实在没人敢相信我能把拳打会。因此老师只叫我站在后面跟大家比划比划。人家花一周就学会 24 式太极拳。我竟学了两个月。但我下决心坚持学，一年之内居然又学会了 36 式，118 式太极拳和太极刀，太极剑等套路。

过去由于多病，说话又不清，没有一个单位招我做工。但学拳一年后，身体健康了，反应力，理解力增强了，能与人较流利的交流，于是重庆低压阀门厂便招我当工人。当我第一次领到工资时，我真说不出的高兴。我都被幸福窒息了。我跑到公园对老师说："我有工作了"！老师和同学们都为我高兴。

至今我已打了 8 年拳了，手早已不痉挛了，嘴不无故扭动了，头也不左右乱摇了，说话也了流畅了。以前是彻夜不眠，现在一上床就可睡熟，以前走路蹒跚，象个老头，现在可迈开大步走，象个年轻人。我还学会了太极推手。有些同龄人还推不过我呢！经过数年的锻炼，我的智力，记忆，接受力较过去大为提高，由发呆变得活泼，但我口齿还不如常人清楚。我还需要坚持不懈地练下去，使我能更健康。

我有了自食其力的能力，使我能自强不息，也使我变得聪明了。没有太极拳，我永远只能靠人养活。

太极拳—让我终于找到了工作！

14. Joan's Taijiquan Story Joan 练太极拳的故事

By Joan White, LADC（执照酒精和药物顾问）

I was lucky to begin learning Taijiquan from Dr. He in 2004. Since then, I have experienced its many benefits including better sleep, more energy and improved mood. I feel better than I did 20 years ago! I have fewer aches & pains and I completed menopause with ease. I even lost weight!

I was delighted to discover Taijiquan is not only good for your physical health but also brain health. My mother and grandmother suffered from Alzheimer's, so I was particularly drawn to Taijiquan's success in preventing it.

For me, the greatest benefit of this practice is emotional. Before I learned Taijiquan, I worried about everything, all the time. It was a habit I didn't even know I had. I learned from Dr. He that with Taijiquan "joy replaces worry". This is so true, and it changed my life. I could put all the energy I used to worry into more worthy pursuits.

I was so inspired that I began to share it with others. I knew Taijiquan could help so many people, including those dealing with alcoholism and other addictions. Often these people have lost much of what brought them joy; I hoped Taijiquan could help. I lost 3 brothers to alcoholism before I discovered Taijiquan. I decided to go back to school to become a Licensed Alcohol and Drug Counselor (LADC) in order to share this treasure with those suffering from addiction.

In the five years since I graduated, I have shared Taijiquan with many patients in treatment. After practicing Taijiquan for 1 week, I asked my patients: "Do you think Taijiquan could help your recovery? And How?" Here are a few of their answers...

" Oh yes! I haven't slept this good in years." -CM, age 55

" I can learn with my friends; we can practice instead of drinking." -SD, age 23

"I wish I learned this years ago I don't think I would have so many issues now." -TN, age 38

"I have a problem with stinky thinking. This really helps", -KH, age 42

"My knees are bad so I can't run to relieve stress like I used to. Taijiquan calms me down." -GP, age 28

"For some reason, I always laugh while I'm doing it! I don't know why, but it's great. I haven't laughed in a long time." -AM, age 47

I am honored to share this treasure with others. It changed my life and I hope the same for my patients and anyone suffering from addiction.

我很幸运从 2004 年开始跟随何医生学习太极拳。从那时起，我体验到了它的许多好处，包括更好的睡眠，更多的精力和改善情绪。我感觉身体比 20 年前好多了！我有更少的疼痛和我的更年期轻松完成。我甚至减肥了！

我很高兴地发现太极拳不仅对身体健康有益，而且对大脑健康也有好处。我的母亲和祖母都患有阿尔茨海默病，所以我特别被太极拳在预防阿尔茨海默病方面的成功所吸引。

对我来说，这种做法的最大好处是情感上的。在我学习太极拳之前，我担心一切，每时每刻！我甚至都不知道自己有这个习惯。我从何医生那里学到了打太极拳可以"快乐代替烦恼"。这是真的，它改变了我的生活。我可以把我过去担心的精力全部投入到更有价值的追求中。

我深受鼓舞，开始与他人分享。我知道太极拳可以帮助很多人，包括那些处理酗酒和其他成瘾。这些人往往失去了很多曾经带给他们快乐的东西；我希望太极拳能帮上忙。在我练习太极拳之前我有三个兄弟死于酗酒。我决定回到学校，成为一名有执照的酒精和药物顾问 (LADC)，以便与那些上瘾的人分享这一财富。

在我毕业后的五年里，我和很多正在治疗中的病人分享了太极拳。我很荣幸能与他人分享这个宝藏。太极拳改变了我的生活，我希望我的病人和任何患有毒瘾的人也如此。

练习太极拳一周后，我问他们："你认为太极拳能帮助你吗？"以下是他们的一些回答：

55 岁的 CM 答道："哦，是的！我已经很多年没睡过这么好的觉了。"

23 岁的 SD 答道："我可以和朋友们一起学习，我们可以练习（太极拳）了，而不是喝酒了。"

38 岁的 TN 答道："我希望我几年前就学会了（太极拳），我想我现在就不会有这么多问题了。"

42 岁的 KH 答道："以往我的想法有点糟糕。太极拳真的很有帮助。"

42 岁的 KH 岁答道："我有一个讨厌思考的毛病，而（太极拳）它真的对我思考有很帮助。"

28 岁的 GP 答道"我的膝盖不好，所以我不能像以前那样通过跑步来缓解压力。但是太极拳能让我冷静下来。"

47 岁的 AM 答道"不知道为什么，我练拳的时候总是要笑！但这很好，我已经很久没有笑过了。"

15. Depression and Anxiety Attacks
抑郁和焦虑发作

By Andrew Ensign

I have had chronic depression since I was a child, though I did not get diagnosed until I was an adult. I never really had a way to deal with it, though my parents found therapists for me when I was young to whom I went occasionally. Symptoms worsened in high school and then became heavier in college. I started using powerful psychochemicals. I started drinking alcohol, at first weekly, then when I went to Japan it became several times a week. Then I found cannabis and started using that instead of alcohol. Similarly, I started out just using it a few times a week, then that progressed to daily, frequent usage.

For many years, this seemed to be effective for me, though it was clearly causing some problems in my life. It was not until 5 months after the coronavirus pandemic that things became untenable, and I had a 3-day panic attack that was one of the worst experiences of my entire life. I weaned off cannabis, and after several months of intensive therapy I came to realize what was missing in my life was something I already knew: Taijiquan.

You see, Dr. Xinrong He had invited me to interpret for her and help her teach Taijiquan 5 years earlier, and of course, I accepted. I learned the 24-step form quickly with her teaching me outside of class, and I started helping with the Qigong class as well. After a few years, we decided to teach the 118-step form, and it was challenging but also exciting. I wanted to practice it daily, but my depression got in the way. Then, during my therapy program, decided to start incorporating it into my daily routine. At first, I just did the short form a few times a day, then I moved on to the long form. At first, I just did the long form once a day in the morning after doing the short form, but I found I wanted to do it before bed as well. I have now been doing the 24-step form once a day and the 118-step form twice a day for nearly 2 years. My depression and anxiety have gone from being severe and a constant problem to being easily manageable, and I owe a large part of that to my daily Taijiquan practice, as well as acupuncture and talk therapy.

I feel better about myself now than I ever have, and I couldn't have gotten here without my teacher and dear friend, Dr. He.

我从小就有抑郁症，长大后才被诊断，一直没有办法治疗。偶尔父母带我看心理医生。高中时的症状加重，然后大学的时候更重了，当时我开始使用作用很强的心理药物。最后开始周末喝酒，在日本留学的时候每周几次喝醉。后来我找到了大麻，并开始用它。同样地，我一开始只是每周使用几次，然后发展到每天频繁使用。多年来，这似乎对我来说很有效，但是显然给我的生活带来了一些问题。

冠状病毒疫情开始 5 个月后事情变的非常严重，我的惊恐症发作 3 天，这是我一辈子最坏的情况之一。再不能那么下去了，我戒了吸大麻。经过好几个月的强化治疗以后，我终于发现了我的生活缺乏的是我早就学到的：太极拳。

五年之前何新蓉医生请我帮她翻译和教太极拳课，我欣然地接受了。她在课外教我，我很快学会了 24 式太极拳，后来还开始帮她教气功课。过几年我们又教了 118 式太极拳，虽然这些挺难的，可是很有挑战性。学的时候我想每天都应该练习，但是抑郁症太严重就没办法练。在我的治疗计划中，我决定开始把它纳入我的日常生活中，我决定每天打拳。我开始练 24 式太极拳，每天几次，然后又开始练习 118 式太极拳。最开始我只是早上打一次 24 式、一次 118 式，可是过了几个星期，我发现睡之前也想打一次 118 式。到现在已经坚持两年左右了，每天打一次 24 式，两次 118 式。我的抑郁症和焦虑症原本是非常的严重，一直控制不了，可是现在都很容易控制。一大部分原因是由于每天打太极拳，还有针灸治疗和心理治疗。

我现在感觉跟以前是不可比拟的好，多亏我的亲爱的朋友和老师—何医生。

16. The practice of Tai Chi has profound health benefits, physical, mental, emotional 练习太极拳对身体、精神、情感 都有深远的健康益处

By Aimee Van Ostrand, L.Ac. 针灸师

I'm an acupuncturist in Stillwater and White Bear Lake, MN. I started teaching tai chi about eight years ago because my patients weren't moving enough. I can't out needle a stationary lifestyle. I enjoyed the practice of tai chi and practiced regularly, on and off. Tai chi got me through some very difficult times in my life. Teaching tai chi began just as a side gig for me. I learned the Yang 24 Form as part of my Masters degree in Traditional Chinese Medicine. The sequence of movements is teachable in eight to ten weeks, there are a variety of movements in multiple directions, and just enough of a mental challenge to memorize the complete form. It is a Form that is accessible to many and can be adapted to be practiced seated. It is perfect.

Mid-March 2020 the pandemic hit and my acupuncture studio, along with most other businesses were mandated to close immediately, for an undetermined length of time.

Without the ability to provide acupuncture, what was my "side gig" became my primary source of income and my community's lifeline. I realized I still had the ability to care for my community, even without needles. During the mandated closure, I taught tai chi via Zoom every day, Monday through Friday. On Saturdays, I led an outdoor group tai chi practice in the park. As the months rolled by, my studio added other online tai chi classes, such as the Kung Fu Fan Form and a Seated Tai Chi, Sun Style. During a time of isolation and uncertainty, our tai chi community grew to include folks outstate. Being online there were no limits to who could join us. Many came to depend on this connection, even if it had to be safely online.

In Minnesota, being outdoors is more comfortable in the summertime. By fall of 2020 many in our tai chi community were encouraging me to continue the outdoor practices all year round. Being from the Philippines, I wasn't totally embracing this idea. I have to say I wasn't too disappointed when another state mandate prohibited group gatherings, even outdoors. We were back to practicing online and I got to stay warm.

By 2021 the pandemic was running its course and beginning to ease up, however many in our tai chi community were not comfortable rushing back into an enclosed room for group practices nor were they thrilled to practice tai chi wearing a face mask. By fall, the challenge was set forth again that 2021 would be the year we practice tai chi outdoors all year round!

We donned our snow boots, snowpants, thermal socks, hats, and gloves. The group took turns bringing kindling, wood, food, or warm drinks. After tai chi practice, we all stood around the fire to keep warm and catch up on each other's lives.

One Saturday afternoon, after a significant snow fall, our group walked up to our usual platform by the river to quickly realize the city does not plow the snow off the platform during the winter. As any true Minnesotan, a few of us grabbed our emergency snow shovels out of our trunks and began shoveling the platform. We were soon practicing tai chi on the snow, by the frozen river.

I remember another tai chi practice in early January at a park overlooking the frozen, snow-covered St Croix River. Our group was practicing the Yang 24. The silence was randomly broken by snaps and crackles of our blazing campfire. The smokey scent of the wood burning filled the cold air. As we practiced, the winter sun began to wane. Then with very little fanfare, the snow slowly began to fall. It was as if someone gently tilted the snow globe just to see the snow float down. It was perfect.

The practice of Tai Chi has profound health benefits, physical, mental, emotional; so much has been documented and studied. But it is during the darkest, most Yin times that we can appreciate how the practice fully lends itself to healing a community that allows us we move toward the lighter, warmer Yang times.

我是明尼苏达州斯蒂尔沃特和白熊湖的一名针灸师。大约八年前，为弥补我的病人活动量不够，我开始教太极。我不能只用针灸去改变不喜欢运动的生活方式。我喜欢练习太极，也经常断断续续地练习。太极帮助我度过了人生中一些非常困难的时期。最初教太极只是我的兼职。作为我的中医硕士学位的一部分，我学习了24式太极拳。动作的顺序可以在8到10周内完成，有多种不同方向的动作，记住完整的动作形式对大脑是一个足够的挑战。它是一种对许多人都适用的完美运动形式，可以站也可以坐着练习。

2020年3月中旬，新冠肺炎疫情爆发，我的针灸诊所以及大多数其他企业被要求立即关闭，关闭时间尚不确定。由于不能提供针灸治疗服务，我的"副业"成为了我的主要收入来源和我与社区的联系桥梁。我意识到我仍然有能力照顾我的社区，即使没有针灸针。在强制关闭期间，我每天通过Zoom教太极。周六，我在公园里带领小组在户外练习太极。随着几个月的推移，我的工作室增加了其它在线太极课程，比如功夫扇和坐式太极。在一个孤立和不确定的时期，我们的太极社区发展到包括州外的人。在网上，谁加入我们是没有限制的。许多人开始依赖这种连接，即使它必须是安全在线。

在明尼苏达州，夏天待在户外更舒服。到 2020 年秋天，我们太极社区的许多人都鼓励我全年继续户外练习。我来自菲律宾的热带地区，并不完全接受这个想法。我不得不说，当州命令继续禁止集体聚会，甚至是在户外也不行，我并没有太失望。我们回到了网上练习，我也可保持舒适温暖。

到 2021 年的秋天，新冠肺炎大流行开始逐渐缓和，然而，我们太极社区的许多人不愿意重新回到一个封闭的房间进行集体练习，还为不需要戴着口罩练习太极而感到兴奋。到秋天，挑战再次提出，2021 年我们将全年在户外练习太极！ 我们穿上了雪地靴、雪地裤、保暖袜、帽子和手套。我们这群人轮流带着打火机、木材、食物或热饮料。练完太极后，我们都站在火旁取暖，聊天互相了解彼此的生活。

一个星期六的下午，在一场大雪之后，我们的团队走到河边经常练习的平台上，很快意识到城市在冬天不会来这里雪铲。和任何一个真正的明尼苏达人一样，我们中的几个人从箱子里抓起紧急雪铲，开始铲出平台。我们很快就开始在结冰的河边的雪地上练习太极了。

我记得一月初在一个公园，俯瞰着冰雪覆盖的圣克罗伊河，我们的小组在那里练习 24 式太极拳。我们燃烧的熊熊篝火发出的噼啪声随意地打破了寂静，木头燃烧的烟雾味弥漫了寒冷的空气。随着我们的练习，冬天的太阳开始减弱了。然后，小小声地，雪慢慢地开始飘落。就好像有人轻轻地倾斜雪花，只是为了看到雪飘下来。这景色是很完美的。

已经有非常多的研究证明练习太极对身体、心理、情感上都有深远的健康益处。但正是在最黑暗、最艰难的时期，我们才能体会到练习太极如何充分帮助和治愈一个社区，让我们走向更轻松，更温暖的阳光明媚的时代。

17. Taijiquan and Brazilian Jiu Jitsu
太极拳与巴西柔道

By Sikai Yang

My name is Sikai Yang and I'm 23 years old at the time of writing this. My brother Steven and I began learning Taijiquan with Dr. He a couple of years ago as a supplement to our martial arts training – we trained Brazilian Jiujitsu & Muay Thai regularly which led to us always having sore muscles, stiff joints, and random injuries.

At first, I was skeptical of Taijiquan. Wasn't Tai Chi something old people did at the park? Why would I, a young and healthy martial artist, need something that seemingly has no practical value in the ring? It wasn't until I truly got to understand Taijiquan through Dr. He's careful & generous teaching that I realized that martial arts are so much more than just fighting. Dr. He taught us that the spirit of martial arts is rooted in tolerance, patience, strength, calmness, and the ability to withstand hardship. In the process of teaching us Taijiquan, Dr. He has always emphasized seeking stillness in movement and using softness to overcome rigidity. Taijiquan is a combination of wisdom and gentleness, and is a perfectly balanced contrast to the fast and ruthless nature of Brazilian Jiujitsu and Muay Thai.

The principles of finding stillness in movement and controlling the breath have been beneficial in improving my training in Brazilian Jiujitsu. Warming up with Taijiquan before doing more physically intense training is an excellent way to loosen up the whole body as well as clear the mind. Now, my brother and I are opening our own martial arts school. We plan to implement Taijiquan as a warm up in the curriculum permanently so that all our students can learn this art. Not only to reduce injuries, but also to learn and carry forward the spirit of Tai Chi.

我是阳思凯，今年 23 岁。几年前，我和弟弟阳思达（Steven Yang) 已经开始向何博士学习太极拳，作为武术训练的补充—可减轻因定期训练巴西柔术和泰拳而导致的肌肉酸痛、关节僵硬和受伤。

起初，我对练太极拳持怀疑态度：太极拳不是老人家在公园里玩的吗？为什么像我这样一个年轻而健康的习武之人，需要太极拳这种慢腾腾的没有实用价值的功夫呢？通过何博士认真而细心地教导，我真正了解了太极拳，意识到武术不仅仅是格斗，更是力量与智慧，包容与克制完美结合的艺术。何博士教导我们要学习太极的精髓：包容、忍耐、坚强、沉稳、能经受住失败。在教授我们太极拳的过程中，何博士一直强调练太极拳要动中求静，以静制动，以柔克刚，太极拳是智慧与柔美的结合，这与巴西柔术和泰拳的快速和激烈形成了完美的平衡。

太极拳在运动中寻找静止和控制呼吸的方法对提高我的巴西柔术的训练水平是非常有益的。在做更多高强度的体能训练之前，用太极拳热身是放松全身和清醒头脑的好方法。现在，我和我的兄弟正在开办我们自己的武术柔道馆，我们计划在课程中常规地实施太极拳教学，这样我们所有的学生都可以学习这种武术，不仅是为了避免受伤，更是要学习和发扬太极精神。

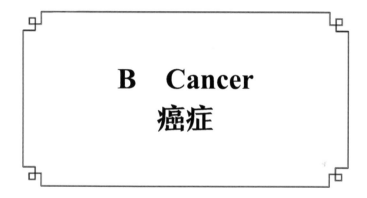

B　Cancer
癌症

18. Second Life 第二次生命

By He Muonrong, Associate prof.

In an accident in 1995, I had carbon monoxide poisoning, and in a coma, my whole body cramped, and vomiting. In order to save my life, I underwent 5 massive blood transfusions, hundreds of oxygen inhalation treatments in a hyperbaric oxygen chamber, and intensive high-dose hormone treatment. But I was left unable to think clearly, communicate with others, and even fall asleep. I, a teacher who taught advanced mathematics, couldn't even calculate how much 1+10 equals, much less work.

Later, at that New Year Party, our president came to me with a toast to celebrate my recovery. After the principal left, I was still holding my glass, and I didn't know to put it down. I was so sad and didn't know what to do. Then my father told me the intense practice of Taijiquan would alleviate my symptoms. Through treatment and insistent practice Taijiquan in the morning and evening, my symptoms disappeared, and I regained my health. I returned to teaching and retired at the age of 65.

In October 2009, When I just turned 65, during a routine physical examination we found a lump in my breast. At that time, I rushed to several hospitals for re-examination. The doctors said that it was not possible to determine whether it was benign or malignant and can only be determined after surgery.

When I finished my teaching course, I was hospitalized immediately for surgery. During the operation, I was still joking, raising my left hand, reminding the doctor that there was a problem with my left breast, so he doesn't accidentally operate on the wrong side! When I woke up, I was already in the ward. The left mastectomy was done, and my doctor told me that the biopsy revealed an invasive malignant breast cancer at the mid-stage.

Even worse, the pathological examination showed it was a Her2 positive tumor, which belongs to the sub-type of breast cancer with a high recurrence rate and requires chemotherapy and targeted therapy to treat effectively. When I heard the doctor's verdict, I felt like the sky was falling, and me along with it. I was in extreme panic, fear, and felt tremendous mental and financial stress. I thought my life was over.

The drug for targeted therapy is Herceptin, which is imported from abroad and is very expensive (roughly $4,000 per injection, one injection every 21 days for one year). In the end, I chose to do chemotherapy, but not targeted therapy, as I didn't want to increase the financial burden on my family. At the insistence of my husband.

The suffering caused by chemotherapy can be unbearable, especially on the first day. Extreme nausea, vomiting, dizziness, fatigue, loss of appetite, and insomnia made me not want to live anymore, and I wanted to give up treatment.

However, with the encouragement and care of my family, I insisted on practicing Taijiquan for one hour every day. I felt that Taijiquan's emphasis on slowness is particularly reasonable, and the act of seeking stillness in movement made my body feel like moving clouds and flowing water. In today's fast-paced life, people are under a lot of pressure. Computers, cars, telephones, and mobile phones are like adding fuel to the fire, making life faster and faster. The slow stretching exercise of Taijiquan helps people return to nature, and makes people feel very comfortable. Through practicing Taijiquan, my mood gradually calmed and stabilized, my mental stress was reduced, and my body became more relaxed, so I didn't feel so tired and uncomfortable. I started to regain my strength, my appetite improved, and I no longer had nausea or vomiting. Taijiquan has helped me a lot in fighting disease! In addition, my little grandson plays the piano for me every day, and my son and daughter-in-law regularly organize singing parties, which gives me unlimited strength and energy.

After half a year of chemotherapy, I survived, and there was no hair loss. The doctor was surprised to see that the counts of my white blood cells and platelets were normal every time I was examined. Then a year of targeted therapy began. Due to the side effects of the targeted drugs on the heart, each medical examination became more stringent. But I finally got through it and finished the treatment.

Later, I went to the home of my sister who is a Traditional Chinese Medicine practitioner in the USA, and received acupuncture and Chinese Medicine treatment every day for a year. I still practice Taijiquan every day. My health and physical strength have improved greatly, and I have also taught many foreigners 42-style Taijiquan, Taiji ball, Taiji fan, Taiji sword, and even went to Hawaii to swim 2.5 kilometers to visit a bird sanctuary.

Since starting Taijiquan, I have felt more and more energetic, and I have traveled with my husband and relatives to more than 50 countries. Every day I on practicing Taijiquan. Additionally, we play basketball and volleyball, swim daily, and teach others to swim too. Among my students, there are 80-year-old swimmers with a life belt and a long rope. I am very proud to have taught the elder man how to swim. I feel useful and my confidence has improved. I have participated in Nanjing college sports competitions on behalf of our school many times and won good rankings in Tai Chi and Tai Chi sword competitions. In the swimming competition of Nanjing colleges and Universities, I have won the top three in the 200m breaststroke three times. On New Year's Day this year, I participated in the art performance of the elderly in Nanjing colleges and universities, and the dance was recorded and interviewed by Nanjing TV Station.

It has been 13 years since I was first diagnosed with cancer. I am 78 years old now, and I am still alive and happy. Tai Chi gave me a second life! Tai Chi is treasures of China!

1995 年一次意外，我煤气中毒，人昏迷不醒，全身痉挛，呕吐。为了挽救生命，做了 5 次大换血，100 次高压氧舱吸氧，还使用了大量激素．我终于活过来了。但是留下了头痛，思维不清，不能与人交流，不能入睡的后遗症。我这个曾教过高等数学的老师甚至连 1 ＋ 10 等于多少都算不清楚，已经无法工作了。那次新年聚会，我们的校长特地举杯来我面前庆贺我的新生。校长离开后，我还高高地举杯站在那儿，不知道将杯放下来。我很难过，不知道该怎么办？

我父亲告诉我，加强练习太极拳，一定会改善症状。后来通过治疗与坚持早晚打太极拳，症状消失，重获健康，又返教学岗位。一直工作到 62 岁。

2009 年 10 月我刚满 65 岁时，在常规体检时发现乳腺有包块。当时很着急跑了几个医院复查，医生说不能确定良性或恶性，要手术开刀才能确定。坚持上完了我的教学课程后，立即住院手术。手术时我还开玩笑，高高举起我的左手，提醒医生是左边乳房有问题，可别开错了啊！后面的一切都不知道了，等醒来我已在病房。

医生告诉我活检是恶性肿瘤，已左乳房全切。诊断是侵润性早中期。更要命的是病理检查 Her2 阳性，属于高复发率的类型，必须化疗和靶向治疗。需要打赫色定（进口药每针 2.8 万，21 天打一针需要打一年）。听见医生的宣判，我好像一下掉进冰窟窿了，感到天塌了，人生完了，思想极度恐慌、害怕、精神、经济上的压力感觉非常大，人整个崩溃了。我同意化疗，不想做靶向治疗，不想增加家庭经济负担。在老伴和孩子们的坚持下，到北京做了化疗。

化疗的痛苦让人难以忍受，尤其第一天化疗，极度恶心、呕吐、头晕、乏力，无胃口，失眠，简直不想活啦，不想治疗了，痛苦、悲观、烦躁伴随着我。

在亲人的鼓励和关爱下，我坚持每天打太极拳一个小时。我感到太极拳强调慢特别有道理，在动中求静，如行云流水。在当今，快节奏的生活已经给人许多压力，而电脑、汽车、电话、手机则更是火上加油，快上加快。而太极拳慢悠悠舒展的运动让人回归自然，让人身心很舒服，我的心情慢慢平静下来，精神压力减轻，情绪也慢慢稳定了，身体也放松了，就没感到那么累和难受了。我开始体力恢复、胃口好转、再无恶心、呕吐，太极拳对我战胜疾病有太大的帮助了！此外我的小孙子每天给我弹琴，儿子、儿媳妇组织唱歌会，也给我增添了无穷的力量！

半年的化疗也就挺过来了，而且没有发生脱发，每次检查白血球、血小板也都正常，医生也惊奇不已。接着一年的靶向治疗开始，鉴于药物对心脏的影响，每次的身体检测更严格，但是也熬过来了。终于经历了死亡门坎的种种考验，治疗结束了。

后来我到了在美国当中医的妹妹那里，用针灸中药治疗了一年。依然每天坚持习练太极拳，健康状况大大好转，体力增强了，还教了不少老外打42拳、太极球、太极扇、太极剑。甚至还去夏威夷游泳2.5公里参观鸟类保护区。

此后，精力越来越充沛，在老伴和亲人们陪伴下开始世界旅行，跑了50多个国家。现在每天我和我的团队都坚持打太极拳、打篮球、排球、每天游泳1千米。还教会不少人游泳，其中不乏既带救生圈又套长绳双保险的80岁老人游泳，很骄傲。感到自己很有用，能够帮助他人，增强了自信。而且多次代表学校参加南京地区高校的运动会，参加太极拳、太极剑团体赛，均获得好名次。在南京高校游泳比赛中，曾三次获得200米蛙泳前三名。今年元旦节，参加了南京高校老同志文艺演出，其舞蹈南京电视台还予以了录制，并受到专访。如今已经过去13年，我已经78岁了，仍然健康的活着，感到幸福，是太极拳给了我第二次生命！感谢太极拳—祖国的瑰宝！

19. Bladder Cancer 膀胱癌

By Er Tong Chen

I was diagnosed with bladder cancer in October 1989 when I was 65 years old. I was very weak after chemotherapy. I felt tired all the time and could not fall asleep at night as well. In 1990, I started to learn the 24-form and Yang-style 118-form of Taijiquan.

At first, I was too tired to do the moves. I could not lower my body or lift my legs. However, after only one month, I felt that my energy level increased, and I could do much better. In the following days, I began to study with Master He Ming, who taught us not only the moves, but also the theory of Taijiquan. The more I knew about the theory and how it can influence the body, the stronger I made up my mind to learn it thoroughly.

Six months later, my health conditions started to improve a lot. I had a much better appetite, and more restful nights, and my energy level increased significantly.

In March 1990, I went back to work. However, I never stopped practicing Taijiquan. Every day, I practice for almost an hour, and the exercise makes me feel energetic and refreshed. For the past two years, the annual checkup of my bladder has shown to be normal. Although I am busy with my work, I still volunteer to maintain the facilities of apartments and repair the heating system for our community. I feel blessed for getting to learn Taijiquan, an art that I believe makes me healthier and more confident in coping with the challenges of life.

Note: It has been Thirty-two years from 1989 since I wrote this paper. He is still healthy today.

1989 年 52 岁时间 10 月我患"膀胱癌"。化疗后身体一直很虚弱，双腿无力，骑几分钟自行车都很累，睡眠也不好。1990 年初开始学 118 式，24 式，起初感觉很疲乏，抬不起腿，蹲 dun 不下身。

一开始，我太累了，不想做这些动作。我不能蹲下我的身体或举起我的腿。然而，练了不到 1 个月，感觉就好多了。以后又经何明老师亲自指导，又多次听何老师讲授太极拳理论，更有学好太极拳的决心。经过半年的锻炼，身体开始好转，睡眠好，吃的多，腿的力量明显增加。

1990 年 3 月开始上班至今。我每天打拳 1 小时左右，打拳使我感到浑身舒服。

两年来多次到医院去复查 B 超，膀胱镜一直正常。现在我工作虽然很忙，负责全院的水暖和房子维修，但很少吃药。

注：从 1989 年至今 32 年了，他还健康的生活着。

20. Recovery From Colon Cancer 结肠癌的康复

By Kathleen O'Donovan, Ph.D. 博士

On December 23, 2008, I had emergency surgery for an impacted large intestine. Following surgery, I was told that I had colon cancer.

Fortunately, I was able to take a medical leave of absence from my position as a faculty developer at the Center for Teaching and Learning . Over a period of twelve months, I focused my attention on holistically healing. As part of that journey, I explored and experienced a variety of approaches to cancer treatment.

Almost immediately, I began to consult with a local Qigong Master and a macrobiotic cooking coach. In March 2009, I began to receive acupuncture treatments from Dr. He. It was during those sessions that I learned she was also teaching Taijiquan.

A friend and I registered for the summer session, which met weekly for 3 hours. I believe strongly that my energy work (*Qigong*, acupuncture, and *Taijiquan*) significantly affected my movement through the twelve treatments of chemotherapy (I experienced minimal fatigue and almost no nausea), as well as my overall feeling of increased energy and a general sense of well-being that I have experienced since the end of the chemo regimen.

I enjoyed being in the *Taijiquan* class. Dr. He and the teaching assistants made the group sessions meaningful and fun. Initially, I found the movements to be challenging in terms of maintaining balance and achieving all the details associated with each of the 24 moves—angles of the feet, movement of the arms, and focus of the eyes. It was a joy to watch Dr. He execute the patterns. To my novice eyes, it appeared as if she were dancing. I feel that by being in the class where Chinese was spoken intermittently and experiencing ancient culture through my whole body, I was learning about the Chinese way of thinking, expressing, and being in the world. My *Taijiquan* world became one heavily populated by intentional circles, focused breathing, and purposeful movements. It was wonderful too, to have Dr. He identify and discuss various acupuncture points during the class, to learn health tips such as 'washing one's nose,' and, finally, to hear about the importance of laughing and maintaining a positive attitude.

Week by week, I found that my body was becoming better able to 'remember' the *Taijiquan* patterns. What I had to learn was to 'get out of my head.' and to trust the wisdom and memory of my body. I believe that Westerners have a unique challenge in terms of focusing on our bodies. Our culture in the United States encourages us (especially women) to deny or discredit the wisdom, strength, and beauty of our bodies. Having taught adult students for more than two decades, I know that it is difficult for those learners to experience new things if they are called upon to perform or to use their bodies in unfamiliar ways. They do not want to look silly or awkward in front of peers. In the *Taijiquan* class, I found both the instructors and students to be patient, respectful, and affirming.

My friend and I registered for the fall session of *Taijiquan*. It was during that time that I felt that the patterns begin to be deeply integrated into my body. My breathing seemed to 'flow' with the movement of my hands, legs, and eyes. I sensed that the movements were becoming more automatic—I had achieved my goal of getting out of my way by getting out of my head!

Since the end of that last session, I have been diligent about doing 20-30 minutes of *Taijiquan* every day. I was given a lovely disc of harp music earlier in the year that I decided to use as accompaniment for myself. It provides a beautiful background in which my whole body can move. Since I have returned to work at the University , I look forward to that time of 'unwinding' at the end of my day. As I execute the moves, I visualize a bright stream of white light moving through all parts of my body. I can almost feel it coursing through my veins and bathing my organs and cells. I can honestly feel energy shifts and 'tingles' as I move through the routine. Upon completing my *Taijiquan*, I take at least another 15-20 minutes of 'cool down' time in meditation.

In my way of thinking, there is a significant difference between believing and knowing something to be true. Without hesitation, I know that *Taijiquan* is helping me heal following my surgery and my diagnosis. I know that it is moving me closer to sustained health. Dr. He is a committed and competent healer. I know that my relationship to her and the application of what she has taught me is key in how I feel and am. My last three PET scans have been completely clear, and I know that the energy medicine that I practice through *Taijiquan* and *Qigong* are significant elements in the management of my health. Because *Taijiquan* is a martial art, I am using it defensively to build up my energy, to create balance within my body, and to support my immune system.

I am SO GRATEFUL for having met Dr. He! I know that her father, Master Ming He, would be extremely proud of the new knowledge and skills that his daughter imparts so lovingly to her students.

在2008年的12月23日，我做了一个大肠的紧急手术。手术之后，我被告知是得了大肠癌。很幸运的，我可以暂时请病假离开我的职位，我是一位大学教学和学习中心的教师。十二个多月里，我一直专注在身心的治愈上。在这个过程中，我调查了也经历了一些癌症治疗的方法。其中一个就是太极拳。

很快的，我开始向一位地方的气功大师和长寿餐教练请教，商量。2009 年的 3 月，我开始在何大夫这里针灸治疗。在治疗过程中，我知道了何大夫也教太极拳。我的朋友和我一起报名了一个星期上 3 小时的暑期班。我强烈的相信我的能量治疗，（气功，针灸和太极拳）明显的影响了我 12 次的化疗。（我经历了小小的劳累和几乎没有作呕）直到我的化疗疗程结束，我总体感觉良好，精力充沛。

我喜欢上太极拳课。何大夫和她的助手让团体学习有意义也有趣。我觉得这些动作是有难度的，比如保持平衡，和注意这 24 个动作脚要动多少度，手的动作，和眼睛要看哪。看何大夫做这些动作是非常有趣的。在我这个初学者的眼里，何大夫如在舞蹈般。我感觉在这课堂中听到断断续续的中文和我经历太极拳，我学习到了中国人的思维方式，表达方式和在这个世界上的处世方式。我的太极拳世界被有意思划弧动作、专注的呼吸，及自觉性的动作所充满，我非常喜欢。

何大夫在上课时会帮助我们找到穴位及讨论其各种好处，这也是非常精彩的，如学习"洗鼻子"的"健康秘诀"，最后，了解大笑及保持积极的人生态度的重要性。

时间一周一周的过去了，我发现我的身体变得更能"记得"太极拳的模式。我必须学会"不用理智"而去相信我身体的智慧和记忆能力。我相信，西方人在关注我们的身体方面面临着独特的挑战。在美国的文化鼓励我们（特别是妇女）去否认或贬低我们身体的智慧，力量和美感。我教了成人学生二十多年了，我知道要那些学生去体验新的事物，如果他们被要求履行或者使用自己身体不熟悉的方式是困难的。他们不想在同伴面前看起来像傻子或尴尬的样子。在太极拳课程里，我发现无论是教师或学生，都需要很有耐心，被尊重和肯定。

我的朋友和我一起注册了秋季的太极拳课。正是这个时候，我觉得太极模式被深深的融入我的身体里。我的呼吸似乎随着我的手、腿和眼睛的运动而"流动"。我感觉到这些动作变得越来越习惯—我已经实现了摆脱"我用头脑"的目标！自从上届太极拳课结束后，我一直勤奋地每天做太极拳20至30分钟。今年早些时候我得到了一个秀美动人的竖琴音乐光盘，我决定从此为自己伴奏。它提供了一个优美的环境，使我身体完全在其中活动。自从我回到大学里工作，我期待每一天结束后放松的时光。当我练习动作时，我想象一股明亮的白光流过我身体的各处。我几乎可以感受到它的运行，通过我的血管和清净我的器官和细胞。在这个程序中做动作时，我可以明确的感到能量的变化和震颤。在练习完我的太极拳后，我会花至少15—20分钟的时间"平静下来"冥想。

在我思维方式里，相信和知道某事是真实的有显著的差异。没有犹豫，我知道在我的手术和诊断后太极拳帮助我康复。我知道它使我更进一步的维持健康。何大夫是一个坚定的，能干的医者。我清楚与何大夫的良好关系和她所教我的东西是我现在感觉很好的关键。我最后的3次PET扫描显示肿瘤已完全消失了，我明白是通过太极拳和气功这些重要的能量元素来管理我的健康。由于太极拳是武术，我使用它建立了我的防守能量，创造我身体内部的平衡，并支持我的免疫系统。

我非常感谢我遇见了何大夫！我知道她的父亲，何明大师，会为他的女儿如此精心地传授给她的学生新知识和技能感到非常自豪！

21. Malignant Sarcoma of the Uterus 子宫恶性肉瘤

By Lianghui Zhang

In August 1986, I was diagnosed with uterine tumors. I stayed in the hospital and had my uterus removed. My condition was very bad, and I was in a coma for almost 6 hours after the surgery. A month later, I was released from the hospital.

Those were the darkest days in my life. For quite a long time, I could not eat or walk; I had insomnia and could not fall asleep at night. I was depressed and felt no hope in life. The doctor wanted me to have radiation therapy. However, I was too weak to do it, so I could only be treated by intravenous injection. The doctor once said that I might only have six months to live. When I learned this, I do not know how many times I cried.

Starting in 1987, I started to practice *Taijiquan* following Master Dai, the wife of Master He Ming. At first, my whole body would sweat even after a short time. Moreover, I was so weak that I was afraid that I would not have enough energy to go through the entire session. Master Dai, knowing my concern, encouraged me with success stories, which lit up my hope of life again. Six months later, the progress I had made surprised everyone. My energy increased, I had a better appetite, I could sleep at night, and my whole-body condition had improved. The regular check-up at the hospital including ultrasound, blood test, and X-ray showed that all elements went back to normal.

Now, it has been five years since I first started practicing *Taijiquan*.

Every day I do the 118-Form and *Taiji* Broad sword for 2 hours. I feel that I am even healthier than I was before the surgery, and I don't even have to take medications. The doctor who predicted that I would live for at most 6 six months was surprised to see my condition. He thought it was a miracle and often uses my case to encourage other patients who are facing the same tragedy in their lives. Sometimes when I think of my roommates at the hospital when I was first diagnosed with cancer, I feel sad for those who have died of their diseases. I wish that they had had the same chance as I did to study and learn *Taijiquan*. Maybe they would be here with me to enjoy life as I do if they had.

Today, I am healthy, in both body and spirit. I save thousands of dollars a year because I no longer need to take several kinds of medication. These benefits all stemmed from *Taijiquan*. Most importantly, however, I am happy.

我于 1986 年患子宫恶性肉瘤，住院后作了子宫全切术，术后休克 6 个多小时，于 1986 年 9 月出院。

回家后，不能吃、不能走，也睡不着，思想负担极重。医院规定要放射治疗，因我体弱，也没放疗，只是采用静脉注射药物。医生断定我只能活半年，我悲观极了不知道哭了多少次。

1987 年开始跟代老师（何明老师的老伴）学太极拳，开始时一练拳就出大汗，体力虚弱又担心学不好，经代老师多次耐心鼓励教导，用成功的故事鼓励我，再次点燃了我对生活的希望。我勤学苦练坚持有恒，半年后，精神快乐，食欲增加，睡眠变好，体力增强了，经 B 超检查，X 光透视，查血常规，结果全部正常。

现在已经 5 年过去了，我还活着，我每天坚持练 118 式太极拳及刀剑共两小时，身体越来越健康了，也不吃药了，西南医院妇产科主任认为我创造了个奇迹，经常向其他病人介绍我练太极拳的结果，当年我一样病情的病友好几个都死了，而我却活得精神愉快，健康，每年至少还节约药费上千元，我真开心极了。

22. Esophageal Cancer 食道癌

By Ma Ruzhang

Prof. at the Univ. of Science and Technology of Beijing

In 1970, Beijing University Third Hospital confirmed that I have esophageal cancer, which had a tremendous impact on my relatives and me.

Since I was young, I have had a strong desire for the prosperity and power of our motherland. But now this disease was going to take my life away. A famous Chinese poem sentence: "He died before he completed his combat purposes, it makes the heroes wet their sleeves with a tear on!" came into my mind and echoed in my ears from time to time.

It was at this time I recognized that life is precious, and I should make every effort to sustain my life and maintain my ability to work. I realized I must not give up on my life. This is when I thought of *Taijiquan*.

My understanding of *Taijiquan* was very simple: I just felt it would be good training for my body, which had become extremely feeble from sickness, and since I made that decision I optimistically and confidently stuck with my plan.

It has been 20 years; I still practice *Taijiquan* and Taiji sword regardless of if it's a holiday or a workday, if it's windy or calm, if it's snowy or blazing. I value *Taijiquan* theory highly and often buy books about it for research and to guide my practice.

All these years I have kept working, not idling away my time. I have also become an amateur martial arts instructor. Taijiquan helped me overcome the disease that signaled death and allowed me to regain my ability to live.

Editor's note: Professor Ma Ruzhang, supervisor of the doctoral candidates at the Beijing University of Science and Technology,, studied abroad in the Soviet Union and returned to his homeland in 1955. In 1970, he was diagnosed with esophageal cancer. He then started to practice *Taijiquan* right after surgery and chemotherapy. It has been 20 years, and he not only adheres to daily work, but also has educated seven doctoral students. He was elected to be an outstanding Beijing model worker for his exceptional work. He is full of energy and is clear-minded; by 1989, he had published 11 articles in foreign countries and had become the highest-ranking teacher in the University.

1970 年我经北京医学院第三附属医院确诊患了食道癌，对我和亲人们来说无疑是极大的冲击，我从少年起就有要为祖国的富强贡献力量，眼看这病魔就要夺去我的生命。"壮志未酬身先死，常使英雄泪满襟"的诗句，不时在我心中泛起，在我耳边回响。到这时，我才感到生命可贵了，我应尽一切努力维持生命和保持工作能力，不能让这一生虚度，这时我想起了太极拳。

我对太极拳的认识是非常朴素的，只觉得它对我这个大病之后，身体非常虚弱的人，会是很有效的锻炼方式，方法既已选定，我便乐观地有信心地坚持下去了。

到现在已经 20 年了，不管是新年还是假期，无论是刮风还是下雨，冰冻下雪我都照样舞剑练拳。我还很重视太极拳理论的学习，经常买这方面的书进行研究，并指导自己的具体实践。

十几年来，我一直坚持工作，没有虚度年华，并担任了业余武术教练。是太极拳使我战胜了病魔和死亡的威胁，重新获得了生活和工作的能力。

编者按：马如璋教授是北京科技大学博士生导师。1955 年从苏联留学回国，1970 年患食道癌，手术化疗后即练太极拳，至今已 30 年了，不仅每日坚持工作，还培养出 7 个博士生，因工作出色曾被评为北京市劳动模范，现在他精力充沛，头脑清晰，1989 年仅在国外就发表论文 11 篇，为全校教师之冠。

23. The Sequelae of Cancer Immunotherapy
癌症免疫治疗的后遗症

By Da Xiao 大笑

I was diagnosed with stage four melanoma. This past Fall, I started immune therapy to fight cancer. Once every three weeks, I would go into the hospital and receive treatments. The immunotherapy caused many negative side effects. I was exhausted and I eventually contracted pneumonia I coughed and had trouble breathing. During this difficult time, I practiced 24-form and Qigong to support my lungs. At first, I would need to rest after each *Taijiquan* cycle. But each day I got stronger. In 6 weeks, my lungs were much improved. My oncology doctor was impressed that he did not have to prescribe me steroids or antibiotics for my pneumonia.

The *Taijiquan* also helped me to relax and sleep better.

我被诊断出患有第四期癌症黑色素瘤。去年秋天,我开始使用免疫疗法来对抗癌症。 每三周一次,我需要去医院治疗。免疫疗法引起了许多负面的副作用。让我患上了肺炎,感到精疲力竭,咳嗽,呼吸困难。在这段困难时期,我练习了24式太极拳和气功来帮助我的肺。起初,我练一会太极拳就需要休息, 但是后来一天天的我变得强壮起来。六周时间,我的肺部得到了很大改善。我的肿瘤医生很惊讶,他并没有为我的肺炎开类固醇和抗菌素。

此外太极拳还帮助了我放松和睡得更好。

24. Highly Recommend Tai Chi now for Anyone Who is Having Surgery. 强烈推荐乳腺癌手术的人打太极

Mary

Soon after a mastectomy for breast cancer and radiation therapy, I wanted to start moving and exercising again. I knew I needed something very gentle, especially for my left side where the surgery had occurred.

I turned to Taijiquan and it was <u>exactly</u> what I needed. The movements, especially cloud hands, were so soothing, both mentally and physically.

I highly recommend Taijiquan now for anyone who is having surgery and radiation therapy.

在接受了乳腺癌乳房切除术后不久，我就想重新开始活动和锻炼。我知道我需要一些非常温和的活动，尤其是在我做过手术的左侧，手术发生的地方。

我转向了太极，而这正是我所需要的。这些动作，尤其是太极拳的"云手"，对精神和身体上都是如此的舒缓。

我强烈推荐任何做乳腺癌手术和放疗的人打太极。

C   Respiratory Disease
呼吸系统

25. Pulmonary Tuberculosis 肺结核

By Yifeng Chen

I am 61 years old. In 1951, I was diagnosed with tuberculosis (TB). I was coughing badly at that time and sometimes there was blood in the sputum. Later, I had two surgeries and the doctor took seven of my ribs out. After that, I got sick all the time, and spent almost all my savings on treatment. My mood was bad too, and I was so irritable that I got angry over very trivial things. For a while, my weight went down to only 90 pounds.

Starting from 1978, I started to learn the 118-form of Taijiquan and Taiji sword. In 1980, under the instruction of Master He Ming, I gradually came to understand the principles of Taijiquan. After that, my health improved a lot. I seldom catch colds, I have a better appetite, and I also gained 12 pounds. Since 1985, I have never once gotten sick. I don't cough anymore. People all say that I look much younger than before. My energy level is much better, and I can walk up to my apartment, which is on the 5th floor without taking a rest, while formerly, I had to stop two or three times to catch my breath. I think that practicing

Taijiquan has helped not only my TB but also my mood

我今年已经 61 岁了。1951 年，我被诊断出患有结核病。当时我咳嗽得很厉害，有时痰里有血。后来，我做了两次手术，医生切了我的七根肋骨。在那之后，我一直生病，几乎把所有的积蓄都花在了治疗上。我的心情也很糟糕，我非常烦躁，常常因为非常琐碎的事情而生气。有一段时间，我的体重下降到只有 90 磅。

从1978年开始，我开始学习118太极拳和太极剑。1980年，在何明大师的指导下，我逐渐了解了太极拳的原理。在那之后，我的健康状况改善了很多。我很少感冒，我的胃口更好，而且我也增加了12磅。自1985年以来，我从来没有生病过，我不再咳嗽，人们都说我看起来比以前年轻多了。我的精力好得多，我可以走到五楼的公寓，不用休息，而以前，我不得不停下来两三次才能喘口气。

　　我认为练习太极拳不仅帮助了我的肺结核，还帮助了我的情绪。

26. Bronchitis 支气管炎

By Wang Shaping

I am a 71-year-old retired worker, who has been suffering from bronchitis, emphysema and enteritis. It was always easy to catch colds.

In Spring 1981, I started to learn the Yang style 118-form Taijiquan from Master He Ming. Master He told us many cases of successful stories of people who recovered from a physical illness by exercising Taijiquan. From then on, his kind and sonorous voice, coupled with his strong body, increased our confidence in learning Taijiquan. I kept on exercising for one to two hours every morning, and 25 minutes at night. After around 100 days of practice, I started to feel much better. Six months later, my bronchitis was totally gone. A year later, the chronic enteritis I had for 40 years went away as well.

As the saying goes, "A man seldom lives to be seventy years old." Now I am already over 70 years old, but my face is still showing a healthy hue. My steps are strong, my appetite is very good, and I can eat half a catty of rice at a time. Every day, I feel that I am full of energy and getting younger. To me, life is meaningful, and the future is full of hope and happiness.

Taijiquan is one of the greatest treasures of the Chinese people. Dear friends, for your better health and happier life, please start practicing Taijiquan!

我是一个年过 71 岁的退休工人，我一直患有气管炎、肺气肿、肠炎，还经常感冒。

1981 年春天，我开始学习 118 式太极拳，何明老师向我们讲述了不少老学员学拳体健病愈的事例。他的亲切洪亮的嗓音，加上健壮的身体，增添了我们学拳的信心，我每天练拳 1 至 2 小时，晚上也练 25 分钟左右，练 100 天后，身体逐渐好转。半年后气管炎基本好了，一年后伴随我 40 多年的慢性肠炎也好了。

　　"人生七十古来稀"，我现在虽已过古稀之年，但脸色红润，步履矫健，一次能吃半斤米饭，我觉得越活越有劲，越活越年轻。感到前途光明，生活有意义，晚年很幸福。

　　太极拳是我们的国宝，亲爱的朋友，为了你的身心更加健康和幸福的生活，希望你也常练太极拳吧！

27. Bronchial Asthma 支气管哮喘

By Yang Changgui

I was originally an elementary school teacher. In 1965, I suffered from bronchial asthma and often had serious asthma attacks. I was hospitalized frequently because of persistent asthma. After taking prednisone, anti-inflammatory drugs, hormones, etc., the symptoms got a little better. However, when I encountered climate change, I could not lie face up, and later I was transferred from a local hospital to the big Hospital in Chongqing Province. I stayed in the hospital on and off for more than two years with no major improvement. Struggling with the disease all day long, I took so much traditional Chinese medicine and Western medicine all year round, and my pockets, bed, and table were all full of different medicines. Until 1979, I was hospitalized at least twice a year.

Due to a loss of strength to work, I had to apply for resignation in 1971 and go home to recuperate. This long-term cough made me feel distraught, withdrawn, and testy. In my daily life, it was difficult to take care of myself. I was very pessimistic and believed my life was at the end of the road.

In the Spring of 1980, I began to learn the 118-form Yang style Taijiquan. In the beginning, I had poor physical strength and was panting. I took two tablets of aminophylline [a bronchodilator used to treat asthma symptoms] every day before I practiced. No matter how hard it was, I wanted to learn Taijiquan from Teacher He Ming in order to restore my health. Every morning at 6 o'clock, I arrived at the park.

I would often take a break after practicing for a while, but with Teacher He's encouragement, I finally overcame the difficulties with faith and determination. Not only did I learn the 118- form, but I also learned Taiji-Broad-Sword, Taiji-sword, and Taiji-push-hands.

Since 1980, my physical quality and immunity have improved, and because Yang-style Taijiquan uses abdominal breathing, I can inhale more oxygen. The severe bronchial asthma I suffered from has significantly improved and did not occur one year later! No more taking medicine and hospitalization. I also became an amateur martial arts instructor. More unbelievable was that I started to work again.

我原是小学教师。1965 年患了支气管哮喘病，经常喘，还多次因哮喘持续状态，住医院治疗，经服用强的松、消炎药、激素等，症状稍好转。但是一遇到气候变化就不能平卧，后由当地医院转至重庆市大医院。住院时间前后积累长达两年有余，效果仍不佳，终日在病痛中挣扎，一年四季不是中药就是西药，口袋里、床头上、桌子上到处都是药，直到 1979 年，每年至少住两次医院。

由于丧失劳动力，1971 年我只好申请退职，回家养病，但因长期咳嗽，每天心慌意乱，性格孤僻，脾气暴躁，日常生活难以自理，内心十分悲观，认为自己的人生道路到了头。

1980 年春天，我开始学习 118 式杨式太极拳，开始练时体力差，喘气。我每天服两片药再去（一种用于治疗哮喘症状的支气管扩张剂），但为了恢复健康，我不管多艰难也准时向何明老师学拳，每天清晨 6 点钟，我准时到公园，常常是练一会休息一会儿，在何老师鼓励下，我终于用信心、决心战胜了困难，不仅学完了 118 式太极拳、太极刀、太极剑，还学会了太极推手。

自 1980 年练拳以来，身体素质增强，抗病能力提高了，又因为杨式太极拳采用腹式呼吸，能吸进更多的氧气，我患的严重的支气管哮喘病有明显的好转，哮喘减轻，一年后再未发生过，也不再住院吃药了，我还当了业余武术教练，更使人难以相信的是，我又重新开始了工作。

D   Gastrointestinal Disease
消化道疾病

28. Cholecystitis 胆囊炎

By Calli Fuches

I went to Dr. He in 2000 because my doctor told me that I had gallbladder inflammation and needed to have my gallbladder removed. I had no stones, but they said that it was "dysfunctional." I decided that I wanted to keep it. I inquired about who the best acupuncturist was and an acupuncture student recommended Dr. He.

Dr. He recommended that, along with acupuncture treatment, I could learn and practice Taijiquan. I have been practicing Taijiquan since then.

Today, thanks to Dr. He, I have my gallbladder with no symptoms. I've learned and worked on many other things since then. My menopausal symptoms have been reduced, and I can sleep well.

The unexpected benefit has been with my mood. For most of my life, I had experienced depression along with seasonal affective depressive episodes. I began taking antidepressants in 1992. Since then, I have gone to psychotherapy, acupuncture, and have started practicing Taijiquan. Today I am symptom-free, and I do not take medication. I have learned to feel and express my feelings while practicing Taijiquan and receiving acupuncture. I am very grateful to Dr. He. Her treatment, as well as her caring for me as a human being, has been curative.

Today, I practice as a psychotherapist. I hold a Taijiquan class during my lunch break. I am grateful for the opportunity to give spiritual food to people.

2000年我去看了何医生。因为我的西医医生说我有胆囊炎，虽然没有石头，但是胆囊功能不正常，需要切除。但是我决定要保留它，不做手术。我询问谁是最好的针灸师，一个针灸学生推荐了何医生。除针灸治疗外，何医生还教我太极拳，从那时起我开始练太极拳。

今天我很感谢何医生，练太极拳保住了我的胆囊，未手术，也已无任何症状了。我的更年期症状也减少，而且睡得好，没想到的好处是还带给了我好心情。在我人生的大部分时间里，我都被抑郁症所折磨，我有季节性的抑郁症发作。在1992年，我开始服抗忧郁药，但在针灸治疗和练太极拳之后，我无任何病症，也不再吃药了。在练了太极拳和做针灸后，我渐渐地学会了怎么表达自己的感受，工作能力也增强了，我非常谢谢何医生！她的针灸和爱心很有治愈能力。

现在我是个心理治疗师，在午休时间我开了太极拳课，我很高兴能有机会把精神粮食送给别人。

29. Cirrhosis 肝硬化

By Chen Jin Hua

In 1984, I was diagnosed with chronic hepatitis and an early stage of cirrhosis. I was put on a treatment that included injections, oral medicine, and physical therapy, which unfortunately had little effect on me. My weight kept on dropping and my complexion was bad. I was fatigued, my limbs were heavy, and when I walked on a level road it was as if I was climbing a steep mountain. My memory was poor, my ears were always ringing, and my mood was extremely low. I couldn't even take care of myself and had to stay in bed all the time. Suffering in this way, I thought that life had no meaning, and I would soon die.

In 1985, when my spirits were at their lowest, someone introduced me to the 118-form Yang-style Taijiquan. In the beginning, just exercising one movement would wear me out. However, my mind would not be broken, and I kept practicing every day for at least one hour. In the end, my hard work paid off and a year later, my health had improved dramatically, and all the hepatitis symptoms were gone. New test results showed that my liver function was back to normal, and the albumin globulin and platelet counts were normal. Now my energy level is even higher than a lot of people my same age. Sometimes, when I am biking around, I feel that life is so beautiful, and I am young again!

我于1984年在医院诊断为"慢性肝炎，早期肝硬化"。吃药，打针，理疗效果不大，体重逐日下降，脸色暗黑，四肢乏力，双脚沉重，走路尤如上刀山，记忆也下降，经常耳鸣，精神不振，生活不能自理，成天卧床，吃不下，睡不着，痛苦极了。我认为生活没有意义，我宁愿死，早点死。悲观，失望到了极点。

1985年正当我投医无路时，有人介绍我学118式太极拳。开始一个基本功做下来，浑身就象散了架一样，但我不气馁，日日坚持练拳，每日至少1小时。工夫不负有心人，一年下来，我的精神变好了，肝炎病状消失，肝功化验白蛋白球蛋白的比例正常，血小板数目正常，体力增强了，甚至比同龄人的体质还好，能骑自行车到处旅游，脸色也红润了，我又恢复了青春的活力，感到生活的美好。

太极拳使我复活，使我恢复了青春！

30. Duodenal Ulcer 十二指肠球部溃疡

By Yuan Mingchong

In 1972, when I was first diagnosed with a duodenal ulcer, I was not really upset about it. I tried to keep a positive outlook and dedicated my mind to curing it. At that time, I chose to practice Taijiquan because I believed that it was one of the best weapons to fight diseases.

Three months after I started practicing the 118-form, my appetite got much better, and my energy level increased tremendously. On seeing the improvement, I had made, I felt more confident than ever and started to make my morning Taijiquan sessions the top priority of my daily life. From then on, no matter where I was, I never missed one day of practicing Taijiquan. In 1980, the GI exam showed that the duodenal ulcer had healed completely. Furthermore, I have been healthy to this day. I seldom catch colds, I've never had to stay in the hospital, and I hardly ever need to take medicine. This turnaround would never have happened if not for my Taijiquan practice. To summarize what I've learned from practicing Taijiquan, I share the following understanding:

First, in order to benefit from Taijiquan, one needs to make Taijiquan a long-term commitment. Don't be frustrated if you are not doing the movements perfectly. As long as you can stick to it and keep practicing, you will see the results soon.

Secondly, one needs to practice under a real master. Simultaneously, one needs to learn some principles of Taijiquan. Having a good teacher, Master He Ming and some books on Taijiquan have sped up my learning process. These two combined will bring double the results with half the effort.

Thirdly, don't rush. There are many Taijiquan forms such as Taijiquan longsword, Taijiquan broadsword, and others; however, I only practiced the Yang-style unarmed Taijiquan. By studying, exercising, and using it for more than 19 years, I have become an expert at it. Therefore, I can practice it freely and perfectly while applying all the principles I have learned. In this way, I have been able to enjoy the many benefits of Taijiquan.

In 1987, I led around 500 workers to Iraq and worked on a project for almost two years. During that period of time, because of the busy schedule, some of us were under great pressure and got stressed out. I started to teach the workers Taijiquan to help them relax. By the end of the project, many workers said that Taijiquan had helped them cope with the stress, and some even learned how to practice the whole 118-Form!

1972年我被确诊十二指肠球部溃疡病，怎么办呢？我并不悲观，思想上轻视它，行动上重视它，意图从根本上清除它，因此我选择太极拳，这是战胜疾病的有利武器，准备长期与疾病作斗争。

练118式太极拳3个月后，食量大增，精力充沛，信心倍增，从此我把早晨练太极拳当成了生活的第一需要，几乎达到了迷恋的程度。无论出差、开会，决不中断，坚持不懈，在练拳中我充分领略到了心旷神怡的滋味。1980年胃镜检查结果，十二指肠球部溃疡已经痊愈，至今未犯过，平时连伤风感冒也少有，担任领导工作20年来，从未住过一次医院，也很少吃药，这也应该归功于太极拳，我的体会是：

(1). 太极拳作为养身健身，治病延年的一种锻炼方式是众所周知的，但贵在坚持，效果寓于坚持之中，无论拳练的好坏，坚持下去都能出效果，当然练的好一些，效果就更大，但不坚持是一事无成的。

(2). 要有良师的指导，再学一点太极拳有关的理论知识，才能掌握好太极拳的基本要领。才能不断地提高水平，我有何明大师的指导，又有太极拳的书，即使在百忙中我也认真学习揣摩，因而得以寸进，受益非浅。

(3). 不要着急。太极拳的形式有很多种，如太极剑、太极刀等；不过，我只练杨式太极拳。积十几年的练习，自然能挥拳自如，纯正大方。体现太极拳刚柔相济的原则，同时也取得了养生健身的良好效果。

在 1987 年，我带 500 工人到伊拉克工作两年多，任务重，工作累，但我坚持练拳，很好地完成了任务，还教会了不少工人练习 118 式太极拳，对减轻他们的繁重工作压力非常有益。

E Endocrine and Metabolic System 内分泌代谢系统

31. Hypothyroid 甲状腺功能减退

By Wang Zi Xin

In 1959 I started to feel uncomfortable with low fevers and palpitations. I visited many doctors and none of them could diagnose my condition. In 1964, because there was no T3/T4 lab test at that time I was mistakenly diagnosed with hyperthyroidism and went through surgery to have my thyroid removed. This surgery led me to have hypothyroidism and I started to have symptoms such as high blood pressure, angina, edema, enlarged heart and spleen, fatty liver, lack of appetite and energy, stomach pain, and discomfort all the time. In early 1981, I was hospitalized for emergency treatment due to heart failure. In the summer of 1981, the factory where I was working invited Master He Ming to teach us the 118-style Taijiquan. I was lucky enough to become a member of the first class. When the class finished, we participated in a Taijiquan contest with dozens of other factories in the district and our team won! This success encouraged me, and suddenly I felt that this was a social activity that gave life meaning. From that point on my vitality and appearance, both changed significantly; I practically forgot what being "old" is, and when I walked, I was relaxed and had a spring in my step.

One year later, I lost over 20 pounds. The doctors had been telling me I needed to reduce my body weight, but I had been unable to. However, through practicing Taijiquan I was able to reduce my myxedema. The weight loss reduced the burden on my heart; I felt more comfortable, got my angina under control, and caught colds less frequently. As long as I exercised Taijiquan I would feel energized that day.

Although the diseases I have cannot be completely cured, I am still happy to have them under control without worsening, thereby extending my life. Before 1981 I was constantly ill, going in and out of the hospital. At that time, I took the hospital as my home. All day long I looked sick and miserable, hunched over with poor posture like I had the worst luck. After starting to practice Taijiquan in 1982, I have never been hospitalized even once. Now my lower back is much straight and stronger, and even my doctor was astonished at my vitality.

For going from being a person afflicted with many diseases to becoming a healthy person, I give the credit to Taijiquan. Taijiquan makes one youthful, improves one's constitution, and improves one's resistance to disease. If you have a disease that just won't heal, give Taijiquan a try. However, waiting until you're already ill to start is not as good as starting earlier to prevent getting sick in the first place. I personally wish that I had learned about and practiced Taijiquan earlier in my life.

我从 1959 年就开始感觉不适，低热，心慌，到处看病诊断不了。1964 年因没有 T3，T4 的化验，误将我的乔本氏炎当作甲亢，在医院做了甲状腺全切手术，造成了我甲状腺功能减退，由于"甲低"，引出全身病，浮肿，高血压，心脏扩大，心绞痛，脂肪肝，脾大 7 公分，疲乏，厌食，腹痛，终日不适。1981 年初还因心衰病危，在医院住院抢救。

1981 年夏，工厂请来何明老师教 118 式杨氏太极拳。我有幸遇上何老师亲自教练，成了工厂的首批学员，学完后第一次参加区里几十个厂的太极拳比赛，就拿个红旗回来，我很高兴，感到这是人生有意义的集体活动，从此我精神面貌大大的改变，好像忘了"老"字，走起路又轻松又神气。

一年后我的体重减轻了 20 余斤。医生要求我减肥，一直未能如愿，如今在练拳中粘液性水肿减轻了，这样心脏负担少了，感觉很舒适，心绞痛也控制下来了，也很少感冒。我感到只要打了太极拳，这一天就有精神。

我这一身病，是不可能全好的，但是能控制住不让它发展，同样能长寿。在1981年前我曾是病危病人，经常住院抢救，那时我将医院当娘家走，一天到晚愁眉苦脸，弯腰驼背，一付倒霉样。1981年以后我开始打太极拳了，直到如今已多年没有住院。现在腰杆挺起，人就换了一个样，连医生也惊讶我竟如此精神。

一个百病缠身的人变成健康人，这得归功于太极拳。太极拳使人年轻，体质变好，能抵抗疾病。如果你有病医不好，请你用太极拳试试。与其有了病才打太极拳，不如早日学会，能减少许多疾病。我就有与太极拳相见恨晚之感。

32. Hyperthyroidism 甲状腺机能亢进

By Ai Xiao Ying

In 1968, I started to suffer from high blood pressure. My blood pressure was often as high as 170 mm Hg and in more severe cases up to 200 mm Hg. I was diagnosed at Beijing Hospital with "hyperthyroidism"; some of my symptoms were shaky hands, irregular heart rate, and insomnia. I had to take medicine all day, and I was very distressed.

Later that year, my health got even worse, and I was diagnosed with arrhythmia (frequently I had an extra premature beat) and had to be hospitalized for treatment. After my hospital stay, I had an infection in my tonsils, which caused tonsillitis; I always had a fever and had to take injections. Sometimes the fever would not break even after more than 10 days of receiving penicillin. I also got a hard pimple on my buttock after multiple injections. With my serious illness being so intractable and all my suffering, my children were often worried on my behalf. Frequently, my children had to take time off work to care for me. I also had to take two or three months of sick leave a year.

In 1982, I started to learn the 118-style Taijiquan and Taiji sword, as well as the Taiji knife from Master He Ming. At first, I did not have enough energy to practice the sword forms after I finished a round of the 118-style Taijiquan. However, five years later, my strength and energy level increased greatly, and I can go through the 24-, 48-, and 118-styles of Taijiquan, as well as the Taiji sword and Taiji knife without feeling tired. After exercising I feel more energetic and comfortable throughout my whole body. If I even skip one set of exercises, I feel that my exercise is incomplete. For the last two or three years, I have had very few fevers, and even without taking medicine, my blood pressure has returned to normal. Lab tests showed my T3/T4 levels and heart rate were normal, and I rarely need shots anymore. After I retired, I was rehired as a consultant, and for the past two years, I have been working eight hours every day. My children are extremely happy with my renewed health.

My biggest reward from practicing Taijiquan is that I can recover my health. I am in a good mood; my family is happy, and I have saved thousands of medical expenses for the country.

我于1968年开始患高血压病，高压经常在170毫米水银柱以上，严重时高达200毫米水银柱，经北京医院确诊又患了"甲状腺机能亢进"，手抖，心慌，失眠，整天吃药，苦恼极了。后来，身体健康状况越来越差，又出现了心律失常，频发性室性早搏，不得不住医院治疗。出院后又常患化脓性扁桃腺炎，每月都发烧，必须打针，有时连续打十多天青霉素都不退烧，臀部都打上了硬结。病魔缠身，痛苦难言，儿女们也常为我的病发愁，经常因请假照顾我而影响他们的工作，我一年要休两，三个月病假。

1982年在何明老师的精心教导下，我学习了118式太极拳，太极刀和太极剑，开始时，练一套拳就气喘嘘嘘，再想练剑和刀，体力就支撑不住了，坚持5年后体力大大增强，现在我每天早上都练118式，24式和48式太极拳各一套，再练一遍太极剑与刀，练完后不仅不累，反而感到全身舒服。如果少练一套，还觉得运动量不够，最近两，三年我已很少发烧，没吃药血压也正常，甲亢实验室化验，T3、T4正常，心律也整齐，已很少打针了，我退休后接受招聘到现在已两年多了，每天坚持工作8小时，儿女也为我的身体健康非常高兴。

练太极拳最大的收获就是使身体恢复健康，让我出全勤，心情愉快，合家欢乐，同时每年也给国家节约数千元医药费。

F Cardiovascular and cerebrovascular disease
心脑血管疾病

33. Sequela of Stroke 中风后遗症

By Dang Fujing

In 1968, I had my first stroke (subarachnoid hemorrhage）at the age of 32. More than 10 hours in the emergency room saved my life, but I was left with serious sequelae, such as epileptic seizures, which occurred every two or three months. The disease not only affected my body but also my mental functions, so I had to quit my job and stayed at home for 8 years.

Just to list some of the countless symptoms:

I had aphasia and lost the ability to speak and write. It took quite a long time to get only a little bit better. I had memory-loss and delayed reflection. I could not express myself properly with the right words. My analytical ability also decreased - I could not figure out the meaning of an article even after reading it several times. I couldn't write, because I always forgot the spelling of words as simple as "No". I had a hard time getting to sleep without taking sleeping pills. I couldn't take care of myself to conduct basic daily activities such as eating and walking.

In 1980, I started to practice Taijiquan with Master He Ming, and it has become a lifelong habit up to this day. Now, all my troubles are gone - I can speak and write normally. I gained back my memory and analytical ability. In the past 10 years, I have become our school's volleyball team leader. Not only am I responsible for arranging the team's daily business, including arranging the travel schedule and boarding, but also for taking care of their emotional issues. No matter how busy it gets, I can always manage to handle everything. All this has proven that I have gained back my health and I can do more than I could have before I got sick.

Sometimes, when I get really fatigued or stressed, I will practice the 118-style Taijiquan, which will relax my mind and boost my energy right away. Other times, when I catch a cold, I will also do some Taijiquan before taking any medicine. And it seems to workbecause I always recover after sweating and getting the Qi and blood moving around my whole body.

To summarize, with my years of experience in Taijiquan, I got the following understanding: First, one must have the belief and commitment and be devoted. Second, a good teacher makes a big difference, so try to find an experienced master. Thirdly, when doing Taijiquan, one should not be afraid of asking questions to make sure the mind is moving with the body. Lastly, it'd be better for one to join a group rather than to practice alone. When doing Taijiquan together, people can be more effective by exchanging experiences and learning from each other.

My language expression ability is several times better than it was in the 1970s. I often forgot the last sentence and the next sentence. I couldn't even ask for directions. Now I can speak at meetings to explain my views, have a heart-to-heart talk, and do ideological education work. For more than ten years, I have led the volleyball team of our school (our school is a high-level volleyball pilot school in Sichuan Province) to participate in winter and summer competitions in Jilin, Beijing, Xi'an, and all over the country. I am responsible for the ideological education work of the team members, and for food, discipline, etc.

After practicing Taijiquan for more than ten years, I deeply feel that Taijiquan and Qigong are one family. It can enhance the physical quality, reduce the cold, enhance the ability to resist disease, and improve the spirit. Now I have no headaches, no epilepsy, and I walk with energy and at a light pace. I deeply feel that Taijiquan has become the first need of my life. It helps me to restore my health.

我是 1968 年 10 月 32 岁时脑中风（蛛网膜下腔出血），在急诊室待了 10 多个小时才救了我的命，但是留下严重后遗症，癫痫大发作，每两三月就发作一次，智力也受到极大影响，只好全休 8 年，当时主要有以下症状：

病后失语，完全不会说话和写字，在很长一段时间内，对病后发生的事都记不得了，我失忆了。记忆力下降，反映迟缓。语言表达较困难，常说错话，想好的东西也说不出来。归纳，推理能力很差，和生病前判若两人，动手动脑写文字性的材料就更加困难，连写"不"字也要问人。阅读能力更差，一篇文章读好几遍才能理解。

我十分苦恼，不会写字，不会说话，连生活自理都有困难。也不能做基本的日常活动，如吃饭和散步。睡觉要靠安眠药，否则连续几天通夜不眠。而且动辄就生病。

从 1980 年拜何明老师为师，学习 118 式太极拳及太极刀、太极剑。学会后天天坚持练习直到今天。我的粗浅体会是：直到今天为止，我所有的麻烦都消失了—我可以正常地说和写，我恢复了我的记忆和分析能力。在过去的十年里，我已经成为了我们学校的排球队的队长。我不仅负责安排团队的日常事务，包括安排行程安排和登机，还负责照顾他们的情感生活。不管有多忙，我都可以设法应付一切。所有这些都证明了我已经恢复了健康，实际上我可以做比生病前更多的事情。有时，当我非常疲劳或压力时，我会练习 118 式太极拳，这会放松我的大脑，增加我的精力。当我感冒时，我也会在服药前练习太极拳，很有效，因为我总是在出汗和全身活动后感冒好转。

综上所述，凭借我多年在练习太极拳的经验，我得到了以下理解：首先，一个人必须有信念和承诺，要投入。第二，一个好老师会有很大的不同，所以试着找一个真正的老师。第三，在做太极拳时，不应该害怕提问题，确保大脑随身体而运动。第四，加入一个团体比单独练习好。当我们一起做太极拳时，人们可以通过交流经验和相互学习来更有效。

我的语言表达能力比上世纪 70 年代好了好几倍。过去我忘记了最后一句话和下一句话，我甚至不能问路。现在我可以在会议上发言来解释我的观点，谈话和做工作。十多年来，我带领我校排球队（我校是四川省的高水平排球试点学校）冬暑假到吉林、北京、西安和全国各地参加冬夏季比赛。我要负责团队成员的思想工作，还负责食物、纪律等工作。

坚持练拳十多年，我深感到太极拳和气功是一家。它可使身体素质增强，感冒减少，抵抗疾病的能力增强，精神好。现在我头不痛，癫痫也不发作了，走路有精神，步伐轻健，我深深地感到太极拳成了我生活的第一需要，它帮助我恢复了身体健康。

34. High Cholesterol 高血脂

By Xi Shengke

It has been two years since I joined the Taijiquan Association. During the last two years, I have been practicing the 118-style of Taijiquan under the instruction of Master He Ming. Even as a beginner, I have already seen the benefits of Taijiquan affecting me.

In the past, I have suffered from high cholesterol, triglyceride, anemia in the brain, joint pain, and other common diseases of the elderly. Due to the stress of work, I felt anxious, and my legs were weak and numb. If I worked too hard, I would have ringing in my ears and my vision would get blurry. In order to change all these things and challenge my age, I decided to learn Taijiquan. Once I started, I practiced hard and paid attention to the coordination of my body movements with my breathing, and I started to see the results before too long.

Now I always feel energized and have a very good memory. Sometimes I only sleep for 6 to 7 hours per day and do not feel tired as I did when I was younger. My cholesterol level went down without taking any medicine. All these changes helped me make up my mind to keep practicing Taijiquan for the rest of my life.

我参加太极拳协会，在何明老先生的悉心指导下，天天坚持练习118式太极拳，至今已两年有余了，虽说功夫尚浅，但却颇受其益。

我已年逾半百，虽无大病，但胆固醇、甘油三脂高，脑缺血，关节痛等老年常见病均有。由于工作紧张，还常出现心烦意乱，双腿无力，脚趾麻木等现象，过分疲劳时还会耳鸣，眼花。不服老的心情使我选择了太极拳锻炼，经过一段时间的认真学习，不仅掌握了动作，而且注意了呼吸及意念等配合，起了立竿见影的效果。

现在我精神饱满，记忆大增，一天只睡6—7个小时，却精力充沛，能与年青时一样工作和学习，未服任何降脂药，练拳半年后血脂降至正常，我决心天天练习太极拳，永葆青春！

35. Coronary Heart Disease 冠心病

By Wang Dayun

I am 80 years old, and I have had a history of coronary heart disorder for almost 20 years. I cannot remember how many nights I've been woken up by severe chest pain accompanied by shortness of breath. Sometimes my heart rate would drop to only 40 or 45 beats per minute. I had to take medicine regularly to keep my condition under control, however, none of these really worked to improve my health.

Since 1990, I started to practice Taijiquan with Master He Ming. Only three months after, my symptoms have significantly reduced, and my sleep was much improved. I no longer must take as much medicine as before. There is a saying that practicing Taijiquan gives you a long and healthy life. For me, these words ring true.

我今年 80 岁了，有冠心病近 20 年的病史。我不记得有多少个晚上我被严重的胸痛伴有呼吸短促醒来，有时我的心率会下降到每分钟只有 40 或 45 次。我必须定期服药来控制我的病情，但这些都没有真正有效地改善我的健康。

从 1990 年开始，我开始和何明大师一起练习太极拳。仅仅三个月后，我的症状就明显减轻了，我的睡眠也得到了很大的改善。我不再需要像以前那样吃那么多的药了。有一种说法是练习太极拳能让你健康长寿。对我来说，这些话是真的。

36. Varicose Veins 静脉曲张

By Leni Erickson

I am 58 years old. Both my parents had terrible varicose veins. I started practicing Taijiquan in my early 20's, and now over 30 years. At age 50, I have ultrasound tests to see how my veins were aging. All the tests showed my veins to be in great shape. I attribute this to Taijiquan!!!

Joints: As I age my joints have a bad tendency to stiffen up, especially my knees. If I do Taijiquan regularly, this goes completely away! No joint stiffness!!! In fact, I rarely have any physical aches and pain and I know that Taijiquan, plus a healthy attitude is responsible.

我已经 58 岁了。我的父母都有严重的静脉曲张。我在 20 岁出头开始练太极拳，现在已超过 30 年。50 岁的时候，我去做了超音波检查，想看看我静脉老化的程度。所有的测试结果显示我的血管情况良好。我将之归功于太极拳！！

关节，正如我的年龄，我的关节有僵硬的坏倾向，尤其是我的膝盖。如果我定期练习太极拳，这种现象就会完全的消失，没有僵硬的关节！事实上，我也很少有任何身体上的疼痛，我知道，太极拳加上健康的生活态度就是原因。

37. Hypertension and Hyperlipidemia
高血压和高脂血症

By Liu Shaoyuan

For as long as I can remember, my health has been a problem. When I was 9-year-old, I was diagnosed with meningitis. When I was 18 years old, I was found to have hypertension with my blood pressure at 150/110 mmHg. I always felt dizzy and had pressure in my chest with heart palpitations. A test I had in 1974 showed that my cholesterol was 318 mg with triglycerides at 170 mg. EKG (electrocardiogram) showed the T wave was inverted, with insufficient blood supply. The doctors diagnosed me with angina pectoris, high blood pressure, and high cholesterol. Every day I had to take tons of medicine, but even so I still felt weak and dizzy and kept having chest pain. Sometimes I did not even have the energy to work, and my mood sank to extreme lows.

In 1982 I started to learn the 118- style Taijiquan. For the first 3 months, I could practice for no more than 20 minutes due to my low energy level. However, 3 months later my body became stronger, and I could practice for more than one and a half hours! A year later, I went back to the hospital and had another check-up and found that my cholesterol level was back to normal. The angina pectoris did not bother me as often as before, and my blood pressure also went down to 120-130 over 90 mmHg. The EKG test also showed that my heart function had returned to normal. Now I only take medicine for hypertension.

My experience has proved to me that "life lies in sports". Practicing Taijiquan not only helped me fight my disease but also enabled me to keep a good mood all the time. By joining a Taijiquan group, I have gotten to know many new friends with whom we can learn and help each other. I believe that without Taijiquan I could never have had the life I am enjoying now.

我从小体弱多病。9 岁时患了脑膜炎，18 岁又患了原发性高血压病。血压 150/110mmHg，经常头昏脑胀，心悸。1974 年在医院检查，胆固醇为 318mg，甘油三脂 170mg，心电图 T 波倒置，供血不足。整天吃降压，降血脂，活血药，仍头昏，胸憋痛，身体状况极差，有时甚至连路都走不了。心情很坏。

1982 年，我开始学 118 式太极拳，头 3 个月每天才打 20 分钟，体力就支持不住了。锻炼 3 个月后，身体日益好转，运动时间逐渐由 20 分钟增至 1 个半小时。半年后到医院复查胆固醇降至 280 mg，甘油三脂降到 150mg.。1 年以后血脂完全正常，胆固醇 200mg，甘油三脂 130mg。心绞痛次数越来越少，血压逐渐下降至 120—130/90 mg，心电图基本正常。现在降压药只吃维持量即可。近几年，心绞痛也未再发作，关节炎也好了。

我的经历证实了"生命在于运动"这一真理。运动不仅能使人战胜疾病，开阔胸怀，保持身心健康，还能广交朋友，使人进入较高的理想境界。没有太极拳，也就没有我的今天。

38. Angina 心绞痛

By Dongsen Huang

On a nice autumn day in 1988, my chest suddenly started to hurt badly. From morning to afternoon, my chest was very tight, and I was sweating continuously. At around 9 o'clock that night, my heart started pounding so quickly that it seemed that it was going to beat out of my chest. I was sent to the hospital and the EKG test showed my heart was palpitating 110 times per minute. I was diagnosed with angina and irregular heart rate. After taking nitroglycerin, my situation got better.

After I came out of the hospital, I started to worry about my future health. I was afraid that I may not be that lucky the next time. I did not want to leave the world yet - I had a good career and my family also needed my support. I made up my mind to gain back my health with all my effort. At that time, Taijiquan was very popular in Beijing, so I decided to learn Taijiquan by following Master He Ming.

Two years later, I found my health condition and energy level had improved a lot. All the symptoms related to the heart disease went away without my even noticing it. Now there are times I am feeling so good that I forget that I once had heart problems. One other thing worth mentioning is that I was diagnosed with tuberculosis in the 1960s, and ever since I have always suffered from problems such as shortness of breath, tight chest, alternating chills and fever, and was susceptible to catching colds. However, all these symptoms disappeared when I started to practice Taijiquan.

When I went to the hospital to have my annual check-up, the EKG test showed that all my heart functions as well as my hypertension level had returned to normal. I have never felt so good in my life. The doctor was curious about what medicine I had been taking. I told him that I hadn't taken anything and the only thing that I was doing differently, was practicing Taijiquan.

I believe that practicing Taijiquan is the best way to keep healthy and improve overall body strength.

1988 年深秋的一天，我突然感到胸闷不适，憋痛，出汗，从上午一直持续到下午，到晚上 9 点多钟心脏又开始激烈地跳动，简直就象要跳出似的。经心电图检查，T 波低平，心率 110 次 / 分钟，确定是心绞痛，心动过速。口服速效救心丸，硝酸甘油药后症状好转。

我很耽心，我若再犯病说不定什么时候就一命呜乎了呢！我想我还有许许多多事未做，课题也没完，我应该对社会和家庭多做贡献。基于这一强烈的愿望，我决心加强锻炼，增强体质。此时，气功，太极拳在北京可谓风行一时，待病情稍稳定后，便师从何明大师练习太极拳。

坚持练太极拳两年之后，我体质大大得到增强，精力充沛。心脏病症状消失了。自我感觉日益良好，在不知不觉中，我竟把心脏病忘得一干二净。出差时的心理压力也没有了。此外，自 1960 年我患浸润型肺结核起，常常出现的气短，胸闷，怕冷，怕热，感冒等毛病逐渐消失了。

在医院复查和连续两年体检，心电图和血脂均正常了，身体完全康复，目前的健康水平是我一生最佳状态。大夫问我，服什么药，从事何种锻炼，身体竟如此结实。我告诉大夫，这两年来我几乎不吃药了。我所做的唯一不同的事情，就是练习太极拳。

我相信练太极拳是全面增强体质有效途径。

G Connective Tissue Disease and Autoimmune Disease 结缔组织疾病和自身免疫性疾病

39. Allergic Rhinitis 过敏性鼻炎

By Murong He, Associate Prof.

I have been frail since birth; I had typhoid and was ill all year round. My mother was afraid I would not survive and found a fortune teller to ask if I would be able to live to grow up. Later, my mother died young, and no one was left to take care of my younger brother and sister and me. Later, I got married and had children. Still, compared to other peers of my age, my overall health is not so good. I had terrible allergies and frequently got colds. My allergic rhinitis was also very severe, so just a cold could make my nose uncontrollably itchy, causing sneezing and runny nose; many episodes ended with a bloody nose. I tried to wear masks or cover my nose with a towel, but it did not help. These incidents could happen at any time, and the whole situation was out of hand. Particularly, the spring pollen made my nose congested and my colds became more severe. Whether I was in classes, eating, chatting with friends, or sleeping, it attacked without any notice. It often made me feel unprepared and distressed, so I did not dare to go out to public places, afraid that I would make a fool of myself. The doctor advised me to check my nasopharynx every six months, and each time the doctor used a lot of anesthetics. Because of the repeated use of anesthetic, my allergies get worse. I also received medicated injections and daub ephedrine to my nose. Anyhow, none of those methods worked. Colds were common occurrences. It greatly affected my study and work, and I was in pain and agony. Simply put there seemed to be no way to work it out. My mood was at its lowest point.

At this time, my father taught me to study Taijiquan; I learned the Taijiquan 24-step short form and 118-step long form. Immediately I fell in love with the sport despite a shaky start and difficulty remembering the routine; but Taijiquan's elegant, soft, relaxing, and effortless movements make people feel good. It requires concentration: you forgot other things as you move, just focus on remembering the movements and routines, and you leave behind all your troubles. You will find that Taijiquan is a pleasure, a very fine thing. I have gradually started to regularly practice Taijiquan, and it's strange to say, but I catch fewer colds. My allergic rhinitis got better with fewer visits to the hospital; I went out with my friends more often, participated in group activities, and my mood got better. Later, I also learned the 42-step form of Taijiquan, Taijiquan jian (sword), Taijiquan dao (knife), Taijiquan qiu (ball), Taijiquan shan (fan), and others. I am interested in all Taijiquan-related sports, and if there is a chance to learn I will not miss it. I also keep up with the practice; I practice every place I go, such as parks, schools, and trains. Taijiquan has become an essential thing in my life. I also participated in a variety of Taijiquan college district competitions; I do not care about rankings; it is all about participation. Once, I woke up at midnight with a sore throat and thought I might have caught a bad cold and drank a little water; by the next day I was fine without taking any pills. Colds and allergic rhinitis finally said bye-bye to me. Ever since I started practicing Taijiquan, I have never been the same I am very happy. I am grateful for life for the benefits Taijiquan gives me!

Sometimes I see friends who have colds or allergic rhinitis and I sympathize with thembecause I deeply feel their pain and trouble. I advise them to practice Taijiquan and become good friends with it!

我从小身体不好，得过伤寒，长年生病，妈妈怕我长不大，还找了个算命先生为我算命，看我能否长得大？后来妈妈早逝，没人照顾我和弟弟妹妹了，以后结婚生子，日子也就那样拖过来了。总之身体没有别的同龄人健康，特别是体质过敏。经常感冒，过敏性鼻炎也很严重，只要一感冒鼻子就不停打喷嚏、痒、流鼻涕，发作到最后是流许多鼻血。带口罩，用毛巾捂鼻子没有用，这个现象随时发作，到了不可收拾的地步。特别是春天的花粉使鼻子不能通气，感冒加重，不管是正在上课、吃饭，与朋友聊天、睡觉，说发作就发作，常常让人感到措手不及，狼狈不堪，因此，我不敢到公共场所去，怕出洋相。医生建议我每半年检查一下鼻咽部，每次要用上许多的麻药，由于多次反复用麻药，身体的过敏现象更加重…，还在鼻子处打过封闭针、点麻黄素、总之能用的方法都没有效果。感冒是家常便饭。严重影响我的学习和工作，我苦恼万分。简直毫无办法可想，心情怀透了。

这时候我的父亲教我太极拳，我学习了24式太极拳、118式太极拳。我一下子就喜欢上了这项运动，尽管开始不太好学，尤其是记不住连贯的套路，但是太极拳运动它那飘逸、柔和、舒展、不用大力气的动作，让人心情愉悦，它需要集中精力，你一动作起来就会忘记一切，只去记住太极拳的动作和套路，什么麻烦事情、烦恼事通通丢到脑后去了，你会发现打太极拳是一种享受，是非常美好的事情。慢慢地我就经常打太极拳，说来也怪，我的感冒少了，过敏性鼻炎，开始好转，去医院的时间少了，我也敢常常与朋友约会，参加集体活动了，心情越来越好。后来我还学习了42式太极拳、太极剑、太极刀，太极健身球、太极功夫扇等等，凡是与太极拳有关的运动我都喜欢，有机会就学习，我还坚持打，走到那打到那，在公园、学校、火车上都打，太极拳成了我生活中必不可少的事情。我还参加高等院校的各种太极拳比赛，不计较名次，贵在参与。有一次，我半夜嗓子疼把我疼醒了，我想可能重感冒了，喝了点开水，第二天起来竟然好了，一粒药也没有吃。感冒和过敏性鼻炎彻底与我拜拜了。也可以说从打太极拳后我的身体，与以前的我就是判若两人。心情愉快极了。我真是终身感谢太极拳带给我的好处！

有时候，我看见有朋友有感冒、过敏性鼻炎，就很同情他们，因为我深深体会到他们的痛苦和烦恼，建议他们打太极拳，与太极拳成为好朋友吧！

40. Scleroderma 硬皮病

By Vibrina Coronado

I have an autoimmune disease that causes muscular pain and has affected my flexibility and balance.

Since I started doing Taijiquan with Dr. He and her associates I have had more flexibility and better balance. I feel more confident walking downstairs and doing things such as stepping in and out of the bathtub. I also do not drop things as often. Before Taijiquan, I felt like such a butterfingers! I now feel calmer and more balanced and able to concentrate on my work. When I have conflicts with people at work, I find it easier to deal with them without getting angry. I can do Taijiquan in my office when I am taking a break from computer work. I got involved due to Dr. He's suggestion and I am happy I took her advice since

I have gotten so many benefits. My scleroderma is improving. In the past, from my fingertips all the way up my forearms, my skin was so rigid and tight that I couldn't pick up a pen. The skin on my face was also taut and stiff, and even smiling was difficult and painful.

After practicing Taijiquan and receiving acupuncture treatments for three months, the skin on my hands and face softened and I could even sign my name. I could also laugh relaxedly, and my face even had some wrinkles! I'm very happy.

Thanks Taijiquan !

我患一种自身免疫性疾病－硬皮症。导致了我的肌肉疼痛，影响了我的灵活性和平衡力。

自从我和何大夫及她的同事一起练太极拳，我便有更多的灵活性和更好的平衡能力了，我感到有信心去爬楼梯和做事情了，如进出浴缸。我也没有像过去那么手握不住东西，常常掉东西。在练习太极拳之前，我曾感到自己是如此的笨手笨脚。现在我感觉到能更平静，更和谐地集中精力工作了。当我在工作上与人有矛盾时，我发现不发火就能应付。当我在工休时，我可以在我的办公室打太极拳。由于何大夫的建议，我参与了练太极拳，我很高兴我採纳了她的意见。

因此我能得到这么多的好处：我的硬皮症在好转，过去从手指尖到前臂皮肤又硬又紧，手不能拿笔，脸部皮肤紧绷，僵硬，笑起来很困难、很痛苦。

练习太极拳和针灸三个月后，手臂和脸部皮肤变软，甚至可以用手签字了。脸上过去没有皱纹，现在面部出现了一些皱纹，可以轻松地微笑了，我很开心！

感谢太极拳！

H　Orthopedic System
运动骨骼系统

41. Helped Me Stand Up Again
帮助我又站了起来

By An Huixian

I was born with osteoporosis, and I often fell and broke my bones since I was very young. When I look back on memories of my youth, I can still remember that I had to stay in bed for months due to these injuries. In 1971 I had an injury again, and this time I hurt my back. The doctor told me that around the back area, several discs in the spine were severely ruptured. I almost crashed when I heard the news because I knew that the spine was central to the body, and without its support, I would never be able to stand and walk again. I was so pessimistic that I thought that it'd be better for me to die than to live and become a burden to my family.

After several months of treatment, I was getting better and was able to get out of bed occasionally. However, I still needed someone to hold my hands or use a cane when I was walking. Then I started to learn Taijiquan. In the beginning, I only practiced one movement–Yun Shou ("Cloud Hands")–which focused on exercising the back and abdomen areas of the body. Nonetheless, I started to see some good results happening to me! The stomach ulcer, which once caused my stomach to start bleeding in 1975, never bothered me again. After I could walk without a cane, I began to learn the 118-form. Several years later, I totally recovered, and nobody could tell that my back problem had almost forced me to stay in a wheelchair for the rest of my life. It is Taijiquan that gave me another chance to stand up!

Life lies in motion. I am 78 years old now and I have never thought of stopping learning and exercising. I believe that by following what Master He Ming taught me, I can always keep a healthy body.

我从小就患了严重的骨质疏松症，幼年起即常常跌跤，非撕裂即骨折，常因多处骨折卧床不起而痛苦不堪。1971 年 58 岁又不慎跌伤腰，医生告诉我，脊柱上有几个椎间盘严重断裂。当我听到这个消息时，我差点摔倒了。我卧床不能动。当时思想压力颇大，我想腰椎是全身的支柱，腰椎折断了，身体无以支撑，成了残废人，不如死了干净，免得自己受罪，又连累家人，悲观失望到了极点。后经治疗，有些好转，逐步能起床，但需要有人搀扶或拄着手杖才能走路。在此期间，我开始练习太极拳中的云手动作，通过此动作练习腰部及腹腔的活动，受到了比较显著的效果。1975 年我曾因胃溃疡大出血，练拳后溃疡再也没犯过，效果出乎意料地好。

在我能丢掉手杖走路以后，又开始学习 118 式杨式太极拳，通过数年锻炼，我由卧床不动的残废人变成能自由行动的正常人，这全靠练太极拳。是太极拳给了我新生的力量，是太极拳使我重新站了起来。几年后，我完全康复了，没有人能知道我的背部问题几乎让我不得不在轮椅上度过余生。是太极拳给了我一个站起来的机会！

近又得何明老师进一步指点，纠正我动作，并教我正确的配合呼吸的方法，使我在练拳时进一步做到肢体舒展，心胸开阔，开始体会到意念，动作和呼吸相结合的重要性，我深信遵照何老的方法，坚持不懈地作下去，定会收到更大的功效。

生命在于运动，我今年已 78 岁了，仍要不断学习，不断练习太极拳，使身体更加健康。

42. Herniated Disc 椎间盘脱出

By James Postighlione

It is a great pleasure to write this brief note for the Taijiquan book. I have been studying Yang-style Taijiquan for over 20 years and teaching for the last 5 years. I first studied the short form, then the long form (154 posture set), which I prefer.

Taijiquan has enriched my life a great deal by improving my health, reducing tension, and connecting my body, mind, and spirit. Taijiquan and Chinese medicine have helped me through several serious injuries and illnesses.

Through Taijiquan and acupuncture, I recovered fully from a herniated disk injury, fragmented vertebral body, and avoided fusion surgery that was recommended by Western Medicine. The increased blood flow and coordinated, fluid movement of Taijiquan helped me recover from injury and increase vitality, reducing and reversing the damage done by injury and age.

在太极拳书上写一个小文章，这是我的荣幸。我学杨式太极拳超过 20 年，教拳已 5 年，我先学的 24 式，后又学的 154 式，我很喜欢太极拳。

太极拳给我许多好处，太极拳流畅的动作可增强血液循环，可以减少身体受伤程度及身体的老化。它帮助我健康，精气神合一。

我曾有过严重的受伤，椎间盘突出，椎体有碎片，腰部疼痛，通过太极拳和针灸中药帮助，使我减轻了病痛，受伤部位完全康复，不需要西医大夫建议的椎体融合手术。

43. Chronic Back Pain 慢性背痛

Dr, Wu Jin MD

I really enjoyed the time spent with Dr. He practicing Tai-chi in the past years.

In those days I was suffering from chronic back pain, The Tai Chi helped improve the strength of my back muscle and ligaments, relieved my chronic pain, and made me gradually become stronger and healthier.

As an aerobic exercise, it provides extensive relaxation for my mental exhaustion. especially when I experienced fatigue, anxiety, or insomnia, Tai-Chi exercise appears to be an amazing power, leading me to a feeling of peace or happiness.

Moreover, I found a wonderful friend, Dr. He, as my teacher in Tai-chi class, She and I go way back, we've been friends since the first session of class. With her encouragement, I learn to keep a better balance in life with more optimistic and considerate way. One of Dr. He's students—Wu Jin.

我真的很享受和何医生练习太极拳的时光

在那些我遭受慢性背痛的日子里，太极帮助改善了我的背部肌肉和韧带的力量，缓解了我的慢性疼痛，让我逐渐变得更强壮、更健康。

作为一种有氧运动，它能使我疲惫的精神彻底放松。特别是当我感到疲劳、焦虑或失眠时，太极运动似乎是一种惊人的力量，能带给我一种平静或幸福的感觉。

此外，我还找到了一个很好的朋友——何医生，作为太极班的老师，她和我一起工作，我们从第一次上课开始就成为了朋友。在她的鼓励下，我学会了用更乐观和善解人意的方式来保持更好的平衡生活。

何医生的学生之一吴晶。

44. Herniated Disc 椎间盘脱出

By Dr Xinrong He 中医博士

30 years ago, my friend was riding a bicycle with me in the back seat. We were enjoying the fun of the high speed when, suddenly, I was thrown out of the seat and hit the rocky street. Immediately, I could feel an unbearable sharp pain coming from my back. I was sent to the emergency room that day, and the X-ray I took thereafter showed that the discs L4, L5, and S1 of my spine were out of place. The doctor recommended that I should have surgery right away, however to me, having surgery was the last thing I wanted to do.

I always think that the body my parents gave me is like a machine, of which each part has its unique function. I did not want to break the balance of my body as being a whole piece and decided not to take the doctor's recommendation. I then thought that maybe I could try some alternative methods to help myself recover from the back injury, and Taijiquan was the first thing that came to my mind.

For the first month, I did nothing but lie in bed, resting and relaxing. I went for acupuncture and tuina (a Traditional Chinese Medicine form of physical therapy), and had an herbal formula. I went back to work after the first month, and it was also during this time I began to practice Taijiquan. Before the accident, it took me no effort to lower my body very deep, however, I could only stand the moves when I first started. At first, my energy could only get me through 10 minutes, but gradually I could practice for 15 minutes, then 20··· Meanwhile, I continued going for acupuncture and taking herbal tea. In the 3rd month, I could practice Taijiquan for 30 minutes without taking a rest.

After the accident, this shooting pain in my back always went down to my ankles, sometimes with a burning sensation. Six months after I began practicing Taijiquan, the pain disappeared in my back and stopped shooting down to my lower body. For the next 30 years, my back never bothered me again.

One day when my husband and my son were working on the roofing, I helped them throw the tiles. I constantly bent over repeatedly to help them throw tiles to the roof and worked all day. Towards the end, I began to worry that my back might hurt again. However, the pain did not come back at all. It was that time when I finally believe that the herniated disc problem I had before had totally recovered. My back now is as good as it was before that accident.

I believe that for no reason will I ever stop practicing Taijiquan, since it is such a good exercise that will benefit both my body and my spirit

30 年前，我的朋友骑自行车，我坐在后座上。我们正在享受高速行驶的乐趣，突然间，我从座位上被甩了出去，背部撞在了石头铺成的街道上。我立刻感到背部一阵难以忍受的剧痛。那天我被送进了急诊室，X 光片显示我的 L4、L5 和 S1 椎间盘突出。医生建议我马上做手术，但对我来说，手术是我最不愿意做的事。

我一直认为父母给我的身体就像一台完整的机器，每个部分都有自己独特的功能。我不想破坏我的身体的平衡，所以决定不接受医生的建议。然后我想，也许我可以尝试一些替代的方法来帮助自己的背部，太极拳是我想到该做的第一件事。

第一个月，我什么也没做，只是躺在床上休息和放松。我做了针灸和推拿，用了中药。一个月后我就回去工作了，也是在这段时间里我开始练习太极拳。在事故发生前，我身体可以毫不费力地蹲的很低，但现在练习太极拳时，我只能站着练习。起初，我只能撑过 10 分钟，但渐渐地，我可以慢慢加到 20 分钟 / 每天，第三个月每天可以练 30 分钟。事故发生后，背部的疼痛一直延续到脚踝，有时还伴有灼烧感。在我练习太极拳六个月后，背部疼痛消失，并不再向踝部放射。

在接下来的 30 年里，我的背痛再也没有困扰过我。有一天，我丈夫和儿子在屋顶上换瓦片，我不断地反复弯腰，帮他们扔瓦片到屋顶，干了一整天。后来，我还担心我的背可能会再次疼起来。然而，疼痛根本没有发生。

我相信我没有理由停止练习太极拳，因为这是一种很好的锻炼，有利于我的身体和精神。

45. Fibromyalgia 纤维肌痛

By Melisa Higgins

My experience with Taijiquan thus far has been short yet profound. Eight years ago, the car accident hurt me, I had many symptoms, and Systemic pain and weakness, which greatly restricted the exercise I used to like. Finally, fibromyalgia was diagnosed last fall.

I have found that with Taijiquan, I can be gentle on my body yet still build an impressive amount of strength, stamina, and flexibility. In just 3 months of consistent practice, I have seen very noticeable improvements in not only my physical bodybut in the stability of my emotions and mood as well. It is great to feel strong again—mentally and physically. I also see Taijiquan as beautiful art that could take a lifetime to master, if even then. But in the meantime, it seems with a little practice anyone could reap its wonderful benefits.

我练习太极拳的经验至今迄短，但很深刻。8年前车祸伤害了我，出现了许多症状，全身疼痛和衰弱，大大地限制了我曾经喜欢的运动。最后去年秋天我被诊断有纤维肌痛症。

我发现练习太极拳能使身体更柔和，但同时能建立令人钦佩的力量，耐力和灵活性。练习短短3个月，我就看到很明显的改善，不仅对我的身体好，也能稳定我的情绪和心情。很高兴能再次感到在心智和身体上的强壮。我认为太极拳是美丽的艺术，需要用一辈子去精通。与此同时，似乎只要花心思去练习，任何人都可以享受到太极拳美妙的好处。

46. Kneecap Injury & Torn Ligaments 膝关节损伤和韧带撕裂

By Amber Johnson

Taijiquan's slow graceful manner and how the posture's flow into the next helped me with my knee's healing process, which I had injured about 8 months prior (Damaged the kneecap and tore ligaments etc.). Over time with daily practice, I noticed that Taijiquan started to improve my physical condition by increasing my muscle strength, flexibility, and range of motion. My knee started looking and functioning more like a knee again! Of course, when I first started, I had some discomfort because I would experience pain now and then depending on the pose we were learning. I took it at my own pace and did notice a difference by the end of class that the pain had decreased.

Another thing I noticed throughout the trimester is that my sleep had improved. With better sleep, naturally, my mood and energy improved. I defiantly can see how Taijiquan not only benefits a person physicallybut mentally also.

I enjoyed it when we not only focus on movements but also incorporated breathing. This combination created a state of relaxation. I looked forward to Wednesdays because in class I would let my stress, anxiety, and any tension seep out of me by focusing on the present and the movements. The teacher's lightheartedness, jokes, self-massages, and stories made it even more enjoyable.

I didn't know that just Taijiquan could so benefit so many people in different mental and physical situations.

太极拳以缓慢优雅的方式以及姿势，帮助了我的膝盖愈合。我受伤约 8 个月了（膝盖骨受伤和韧带撕裂等），经过一段时间的每日练习太极拳，我发现它开始改善我的身体状况，增加我肌肉的力量和其范围的灵活性。我的膝盖和功能看起来像一个膝盖了。当然，当我第一次开始学习太极拳的时候，我有一些不适，因为我偶尔会感到疼痛，这取决于我们正在学习的姿势。后来我按照自己的节奏学习，在课程结束时确实注意到疼痛减轻了。

另一件事，我注意到经过了三个月的太极拳练习，我的睡眠改善了，有了更好的睡眠，我的心情和精力自然有所改善。我明确的看到了太极拳不止对一个人的身体好，对心智也好。

我喜欢练太极拳时不仅注重动作，也配合呼吸。这种结合创造了一个放松的状态。我期待星期三上课日子的到来，因为在课堂上，会让我所有的压力，焦虑和紧张的状态释放出来，通过专注地去做动作，加上老师的轻松态度，讲笑活，自我按摩，讲故事，使课程就更有趣了。

太极拳真是能让许多人在心理和身体上都受益！

47. Frozen Shoulder 肩周炎

By Carolyn Tapia

I began studying Taijiquan with Dr. Xinrong He approximately 8 years ago in 1997, and I return periodically for review classes. When I practice Taijiquan on a regular basis I notice many benefits such as greater strength in my back and legs and improved balance, coordination, and flexibility. I also feel more relaxed and serene during and after playing Taijiquan. On more than one occasion I started Taijiquan with a headache stemming from chronic neck pain and by the end of the class, I was free of pain.

The most remarkable experience I had with Taijiquan was approximately 3 years ago when I developed a "frozen" shoulder as a result of a rotator cuff injury. The range of motion in my right arm and shoulder was severely restricted, interfering with various daily activities. The physical therapist gave me a poor prognosis due to my age (over 50). Neither physical therapy alone nor osteopathic adjustments were beneficial and although acupuncture relieved the pain in the shoulder, it remained "frozen" until I started moving it slowly and gently in daily Taijiquan exercise. Slowly my range of motion returned to normal, and I resumed my regular activities including yoga, bicycling, and gardening.

I am grateful for the many gifts I continue to receive from Taijiquan. I am especially grateful to Dr. He as my physician and Taijiquan teacher for her very generous spirit and all I have learned from her.

在大概 8 年前的 1997 年，我开始向何新蓉大夫学太极拳，我也常回来参加复习课程。当我定期练太极拳，我发现有许多好处，我的背和腿更有力了，平衡和柔软度变好了。我觉得打太极拳，让我更放松和平和，有时候我有因慢性颈痛引起的头痛，练了太极拳之后就不痛了。

太极拳最显著的功效是在大约三年前，因我肩关节受伤引起"冰冻"肩周炎，肩膀僵硬，我右肩和手臂活动范围大大减少，影响许多日常活动。我的理疗师认为我的预后很差，因为我已超过 50 岁了。康复和整骨治疗对我没有帮助，虽然针灸缓解了肩膀的疼痛，但是它依然是"冻结"状态。但是太极拳帮助我减轻疼痛，我慢慢地轻轻地每天练太极拳，就不僵硬了。慢慢地渐渐地我肩膀的活动范围恢复正常，而我也能开始做平常的活动，像瑜伽、骑自行车、整理花园，

我很感谢太极拳给我许多的礼物。我特别要谢谢何大夫作为我的医生和太极拳老师，感谢她非常慷慨的精神和我从她身上学到的一切。

I   Taijiquan and Mental Health 太极拳与心理健康

48. Taijiquan Has Made Me More Inwardly Focused.
太极让我更注重内心意识

Dr. Jim Stevenson MD

Taijiquan is an ancient Chinese form of yoga. All action, believe it or not, is preceded by thought. of all heritages have realized this truth. The Bible says, "Blessed are the pure in heart for they shall see God." The mystics in all traditions realized this. Thought precedes action. Tai Chi is thus a discipline enabling one to go beyond the world of thought to a world of positive action, both physically and mentally. Taijiquan that I tried to pass on to my patients.

Taijiquan has made me more inwardly focused.

太极拳是中国最古老的一种瑜伽形式。信不信由你，一切行动都以思想为先。历代圣贤都认识到了这个真理。圣经说："纯洁的人是有福的，因为他们必看见神。"传统中的圣贤们都意识到：思想先于行动。因此，太极是一种学科，使一个人能够超越思想的世界，进入一个身体上和精神上都积极行动的世界。太极创造了一种内在的生活方式，我试图把它传递给我的病人。

太极让我更注重内心意识。

49. Got Married 我结婚了

By E.T. Nancy

I have a few health problems. The main ones are bipolar disorder, fibromyalgia, ulcerative colitis, asthma, arthritis, and mild head injury. There was a time when I was very sick and depressed. I lost interest in everything around me; I remember going to see Dr. He for acupuncture, and I couldn't open her door to get into the clinic. I didn't even have the strength to life a cup of tea. I felt very humiliated about not having any energy, so I became depressed.

I'm not sure when I took my first Taijiquan lesson from Dr. He. My best guess is 1998. I had a difficult time learning the moves because of my memory problems. Dr. He was very patient with me and would practice with me often. She even took time out from her busy acupuncture schedule to review Taijiquan with me at her office. Sometimes we would go out in the hallway with her assistant Cary and practice Taijiquan. We did get some funny looks from folks passing by.

One time when I took the Taijiquan class, Dr. He's father, Master Ming He, was teaching it with her. I enjoyed getting to know him, and he was an inspiring example. I could tell that practicing Taijiquan had kept him healthy. He looked like a sweet little old man, but he was surprisingly strong. I had to quit practicing the defensive moves with him, because he would hurt me sometimes! I think he didn't realize how much force he put into the moves. I also remember doing Taijiquan with him outside Dr. He's house at a party. He would go over moves repeatedly till I could do them well.

More recently, my daughter Ann and I took a Taijiquan fan class from Dr. He's sister Mu Rong He. Dr. He and her son Henry were assistant teachers in that class. It was fun watching Henry do Taijiquan fan moves. Ann and I both had a great time. However, Ann learned the moves more quickly than I did. Mu Rong kindly coached and encouraged Ann, which made Ann feel special.

Practicing Taijiquan is one of the tools that help me manage my health. I have been doing well the last few years. I appreciate being able to drive a car, do my own shopping, and have a social life.

I was married on April 23rd, 2005, to a wonderful man named Mike. He also attended Dr. He's Taijiquan class and both of us practiced Taijiquan in the class. Dr. He performed Taijiquan fan beautifully at our wedding, and then we all danced.

I am very grateful to Dr. He, her family, and the other instructor Caryl!

我有一些健康问题主要有双相情感障碍、纤维肌痛、溃疡性结肠炎、哮喘、关节炎、轻度头部损伤。有一段时间我病得很重，情绪低落，对周围的一切都失去兴趣。我记得我去看何大夫做针灸，我手无力以至于不能打开她的门进入诊所。我甚至连提茶杯的力气都没有。我感到很尴尬，因为没有任何精力，我变得很沮丧。

我不确定我是什么时候从何医生那里学的太极拳。我猜是1998年。由于我的记忆问题，我很难学会这些动作。我因有记忆慢的问题，学起来很慢，何大夫很有耐心，常陪我一起练习。她甚至从忙碌时间中抽空和我一起练太极拳。有时我会和她的助理一起在诊所门外练太极拳，很多人经过时，用奇异眼光看我们。

有一次太极拳课是何大夫父亲何明大师来教的，他是一个积极向上的表率，我很高兴认识他，因为太极拳使他很健康，他看起来是个可爱的小个子，但却惊人的强壮。我不能够与他练习太极拳攻防，怕他不知道自己力气大，会无意中会伤到我。在何大夫家开 party 时，何明老师会一直重复太极拳动作，让我能学会太极拳。

后来我女儿和我一起上何大夫的姐姐何慕蓉的太极扇课，何大夫和她的儿子 Henry 也一起教，Henry 的太极扇动作很优美。我的女儿安与我都学得很开心，女儿安学动作比我快多了，慕蓉老师极温柔，总是鼓励安，让安感到自己很特别。

练太极拳是一个帮我恢复健康的好方法。过去的几年我过得非常好，我感谢太极拳让我躁郁症好转很多，我能自己购物，有社交生活，还能开车狂飙。

在 2005 年 4 月 23 日我结婚了！我嫁给了一个很棒的男人迈克。他也参加了何大夫的太极拳班，我们俩在一个班练习太极拳。何大夫参加了我的婚礼，她表演了太极扇，我们还一起跳了舞。

我很感谢何大夫家人和另一教练 Cary ！

50. Taijiquan Accompanied Me Through the Times of Depression
太极拳陪我度过抑郁的时光

By Lao Yang   professor 教授

As the Coronavirus 19 lasted for too long, I lived alone, I became depressed and I wanted to cry,I think I must try to overcome this trouble I want to make my life full, I decided to play Taijiquan several times every morning and evening, Baduanjin, also with massage the Shanzhong point. After a period of persistence, my feeling has improved, I have continued to practice Taijiquan Baduanjin. From my personal experience, I realize that Taijiquan has the effect of regulating emotions. I also feel that my sleep has improved better. I can often sleep overnight until dawn, and no longer get up at night. When I really have a good mood, people will be refreshed.

Taijiquan can not only invigorate the muscles and bones, balance qi and blood, strengthen the body, but also can adjust the mood, improve the quality of sleep, enhance the body immunity, is really a lot of benefits, friends insist on practicing Taijiquan!!

由于冠状病毒19疫情延续了太长时间，我一个人居住，心情变得闷闷不乐，有想哭的感觉，我想我必须想方设法克服这个问题。我要把自己的日子过得充实些，我决定每天早晚多打几遍太极拳，八段锦，也配合按摩膻中穴，经过一段时间的坚持，自己的感觉有了好转，我就一直延续着打太极拳八段锦的练习。从我的切身体会中认识到打太极拳是有调节情志的功效，我同时也感觉到我的睡眠有更好的改善，常常能一夜睡到大天亮，不再起夜了，真的心情好了，人就精神了。

打太极拳不仅活络筋骨，平衡气血，强身健体，也能调节情志，改善睡眠质量，增强机体免疫力，真的是好处多多，朋友们坚持练习太极拳吧！！

51. Practicing Taichiquan Makes Me Healthy and Happy 太极拳让我健康快乐

Zhen Zou
Prof. of Minnesota University 明尼苏达大学教授

I started practicing Taijiquan in 2005. The year before that, it was found that I had elevated reading of the platelets. It was a lot higher than normal. My family doctor thus referred me to a hematologist. That hematologist, a doctor in his forties, originally from India but trained in the United States, was very knowledgeable with rich experience. He gave me two medicines to choose from. I selected one of them, but it was not effective. Instead, it had very serious side effects. After taking it for a month or so, I felt very weak and tired, and had great difficulty even going up the stairs. My hematologist then suggested that I take the other kind of medicine. Fortunately, the second medicine was miraculously effective on me. My platelet number came down quickly, and, within a month, the reading was normal again. Besides, it did not seem to have any side effects on me.

Although my platelet reading was back to normal, the elevated reading of platelet in the previous months had damaged my health, and I was not able to enjoy good health for some time. Instead, I was in a state of so-called "sub-health," and not feeling great at all. Just at that time, I learned that Dr. Xinrong He was teaching Taijiquan at the American Academy of Acupuncture and Oriental Medicine (AAAOM), and I immediately signed up to learn Taijiquan from her. What Dr. He taught was 24 Simplified Taijiquan, which is the most common and most popular Taijiquan practiced in China. Although labeled as "simplified," it was not at all easy to remember all the movements and the sequence of them. To help students learn, Dr. He wrote down the names of all the movements and their sequence from movement 1 to 24, and distributed the sheet to all the students. I knew that Dr. He taught many sessions of Taijiquan. Each session lasted ten weeks, with two classes a week. In the first class, before formally teaching Taijiquan movements, Dr. He told us the essentials of Taijiquan: When you start Taijiquan, put your feet apart as wide as the shoulders; keep shoulders and elbows low; inhale air and put the air below the navel. In addition, controlled breathing should go throughout the process of Taijiquan practice. Obviously, Dr. He combined Taijiquan with breathing exercises, which is exactly what they call "Taijiquan/ Qigong (Breathing Exercises)" in China.

After telling students the essentials of doing Taijiquan, Dr. He began to teach Taijiquan movements. From the second Taijiquan class on, Dr. He would lead the students to review, practice, and consolidate the movements that had been taught in previous classes before moving on to teach new movements. Dr. He is a very responsible and conscientious instructor, and requires every students to do every movement to her high standard. Whenever she started to teach a new movement, she would first tell the students the name of the movement, demonstrate several times in detail how to do the movement correctly, before letting the students follow her demonstration step by step. She also took pains to correct every student until everybody did the movement correctly. As a result, students who graduated from Dr. He's class have very high standard Taijiquan movements.

In addition to teaching the Taijiquan movements, Dr. He also told students to breathe properly while practicing Taijiquan. That is, whether one should inhale or exhale while doing each of the movements. While demonstrating each movement and letting students follow her, she would say slowly, "Breathe – in ," or "Breathe – out." As a result, students were able to integrate Taijiquan movements with breathing exercises. From what Dr. He taught us, my understanding is that when a movement is "closing in," i.e., when the hand(s) and feet are moving towards the body, we should breathe in, which naturally entails accumulating strength. On the other hand, when a movement is "going out," like pushing, kicking, and so on, breathing out accompanies the action, thus empowering the action and movement. Moreover, integrating breathing exercises with Taijiquan movements also enhances the effect of Taijiquan practice.

In addition to teaching all the movements of the whole set of Taijiquan, Dr. He also taught students how to use Taijiquan for self-defense. For example, she showed us how to use the movement of "Waving Hands in the Clouds" to dissolve assault from an attacker and find a gap in the other's defense to counter-offense. In case your hand is grabbed by your attacker, how to use "Apparent Close up" to free your hand. If an attacker rushes to hit you aggressively, how to use "Grasp the Bird's Tail" to pull the attacker and throw him onto the ground even before he realizes what has happened, and so on.

By the end of the tenth week, not only had Dr. He taught the students the essentials of practicing Taichiquan, but also all the 24 movements of it. As Dr. He is such a conscientious and diligent instructor and spared no effort in correcting students' gestures and movements, all the students had mastered the whole set of Taijiquan with standard movements. At the end of the session, Dr. He also told the students to practice Taijiquan 30 minutes every day to attain good health. Moreover, if one integrates breathing exercises with Taijiquan, the effect is even better.

In the final class of the Taijiquan session, Dr. He invited another expert to perform with her "Taiji Fan" for us. The two experts performed Taiji Fan accompanied with music, and their movements were amazing to watch. Throughout their performance, the sounds of "Opening" and "Closing" of the fans coupled with beautiful movements were not only pleasant to watch, but also graceful and powerful that all the people present were fascinated. When the whole set was completed, loud and long claps of hands expressed the students' genuine admiration of the masters' Taichi Fan performance.

Ever since I learned Taijiquan from Dr. He, I started to practice it every day. Before that, I also learned Breathing Exercises (Qi Gong/ Chi Gong), so beginning from 2005, I have been having 30 minutes of Breathing Exercises + 30 minutes of Taijiquan every morning. After several years, I began to feel the effect of these exercises, and I was no longer in the state of "sub-health."

America is a country where the benefits of sports and exercises are emphasized. In 2008, my employer, the University of Minnesota, encouraged students, faculty and staff to use school gyms, and provided free access to gym facilities, including the swimming pools. After trying the swimming pool for a semester, I fell in love with this sport, and decided to add swimming to my weekly exercises. I increased the frequency of my swimming exercises from two times to three times a week, and the distance from 100 yards to 200, then 300, till I could swim more than 1000 yards every time without a break. I did that for more than ten years, and in those years I felt healthier than ever before. In my annual physical exam, my blood picture was much better than in 2004 or 2005. Everything in my hemogram was normal, including the platelet readings, even though I had gradually reduced the amount of the platelet-medicine and eventually stopped using it completely in 2017. As I enjoyed good health, I was always in good mental and spiritual state, and felt happy, cheerful and optimistic almost all the time. I attributed my health and positive state of mind to practicing Taijiquan, breathing exercises, and swimming, believing that these exercises greatly improved my health and enabled me to enjoy life more than ever before.

The year of 2020 came with the Pandemic. To prevent the spread of COVID-19 virus, gyms were closed. In March of that year, I had to stop my swimming exercises, and I have not been able to swim for more than two years and a half. Moreover, due to the bitter-cold winter in Minnesota, outdoor exercise is virtually impossible, including jogging. As a result, during the seasons of winter and spring in the past several years, I was not able to do any strenuous exercises, and my exercises were limited to Taijiquan and breathing. As Breathing exercises has very little movements of the limbs, Taijiquan was my only exercise with movements in the real sense of the word. Owing to the drastically reduced amount of exercises, I was really worried that my health would deteriorate during those years. To my surprise, however, the results of my recent physical examination told a different story. The numbers of my blood picture were all normal! Obviously, it was the result of daily Taijiquan. I owe my health to Taijiquan practice.

An unexpected opportunity even put me on stage to perform Taijiquan. Here is what happened: In the annual production of 2018 for Minhua Chorus where I was a member, we had a men's chorus piece called "The Rolling Yangtze Running East." The lyrics were by Yang Shen, a poet of the Ming Dynasty about 500 years ago. Put into melody by a renowned Chinese musician Gu Jianfen, this song was used at the beginning of every episode of the history Television series Romance of the Three Kingdoms. The version we used had a prelude that lasted a whole minute, which meant that all the singers had to stand still on stage waiting for the prelude to play out before starting to sing. Both the singers and the audience would feel awkward during that time. Someone then suggested that I perform Taijiquan during the time of the prelude. At first hearing of this idea, I was taken by surprise. After thinking about this idea, however, I realized that it made a lot of sense: Romance of the Three Kingdoms was a novel that depicted a period of highly eventful Chinese history; "The Rolling Yangtze Running East" expressed one's broad mind of cherishing the Chinese history and culture of more than five thousand years and talking about all the historical events with a smile; and Taijiquan is a highlight of deep-rooted Chinese culture. Putting the three together was really a comprehensive expression of Chinese history and culture that could greatly enrich this performance piece. After accepting this challenge, I discussed the performance with another great master of Taijiquan in the Twin Cities, Caiyun Zhou and asked for her advice. I employed several movements from the set of Taijiquan which Dr. He taught me, and added several other movements from that master. Together we designed a micro set of Taijiquan that temper strength with gentleness, and I began to practice this set with the music of the prelude. On the day of the performance, all the singers stood on the stage in a row. Up went the curtain, the music started, and I performed this micro set of Taijiquan. It went well. Just at the end of the prelude, I completed the micro Taijiquan, and the male chorus started to sing. The Conductor, members of the chorus, and the audience all agreed that it was a great piece of performance. They especially complimented the micro Taijiquan during the prelude, saying that it increased the quality and richness of the performance, making it much more enjoyable to watch.

Evidently, practicing Taijiquan not only has been strengthening my physical constitution and giving me good health to enjoy, but also enabled me to combine it with art, and has made me healthy and happy.

我是从 2005 年开始习练太极拳的。此前一年，我在年度体检时查出血小板增高，比正常值高出很多。我的家庭医生让我针对这个问题看血液病的专科医生，我的那位血液专科医生是个印度人，四十多岁，专业知识和经验都很丰富。他告诉我，要把血小板降下来，有两种药可以用。在介绍了这两种药各自的特点后，医生让我选择其中的一种。但是第一种药服用了几个月后，基本上没效果，而且副作用比较大，常常感觉疲乏，浑身无力，连上楼都困难。那位印度医生于是让我服用另外一种药。第二种药在我身上效果非常明显，血小板很快降了下来，回到正常水平。虽然血小板降下来了，但由于前一段时间血小板太高，对身体造成了损害，所以那时我的身体状况总是不太好，处于一种"亚健康"的状态。这样的健康状况对生活、工作都不利，必须改变。

就在那时候，我得知何新蓉大夫在美国中医学院开办了太极拳培训班，就报名参加。何大夫教授的是二十四式简化太极拳，这是在中国练习人数最多的一种太极拳。虽说是"简化"，但初学者要记住二十四式的动作和顺序并非易事。为帮助学员们学习掌握，何大夫把所有二十四式的名称和顺序都写下来，发给学员。记得何大夫的太极拳培训班每期10个星期，每星期两个晚上上课，一共二十次课。在正式教太极拳动作之前，何大夫先给学员们介绍练习太极拳的基本要领：起势时要双脚与肩同宽，沉肩垂肘，气沉丹田，而且有规律地运气贯穿整个练太极拳的过程，所以何大夫把太极拳跟气功结合起来了，正好符合民间素有的"太极气功"之说。每次上课时，何大夫先带学员们复习上一次学过的内容，然后教新的招式。何大夫教课极其认真，每一个动作她都要求完全做到位，而且每教一个动作，她都要首先示范好几遍详细的分解动作，再一边说着分解动作的名字，一边一步一步地让学员们做，并且给学员们挨个纠正，直到每一个学员的动作都做准确了，才接着教下一个动作。所以从何大夫太极拳培训班出来的学员动作都很准确、到位。此外，每教一个动作，何大夫都会一边教，一边告诉学员"吸气"还是"呼气"，这样就让学员们很自然地把太极拳的一招一式和呼吸 / 气功结合起来，融为一体。从何大夫的教学中，我理解到太极拳往里收的动作一般都配合吸气，而往外放 (包括踢、打等) 的动作大都配合呼气。我感觉这样练太极拳，往里收的招式能在体内积蓄力量，往外放的招式配合呼气，手、臂、腿、脚的力量就更大，增强了锻炼身体的效果。何大夫不但教授整套太极拳的动作，而且还教学员们如何用太极拳防身。例如，怎样用 "云手" 化解对方的攻势，然后找出对方防守的破绽进行反击；万一手被对方抓住时，怎样用 "如封似闭" 迅速摆脱对方的抓握；怎样借力打力：如果对方来势汹汹，一拳打过来，怎样用 "将" 这个动作顺势将对方一拉，让他失去平衡，对方还没明白是怎么回事，就把他摔倒在地，等等。十个星期下来，何大夫不但把整套 24 式太极拳都传授给了学员们，而且由于何大夫教学认真、一丝不苟，严格要求，在整个教学期间不断纠正学员们的动作，所以大家的动作都很标准。全套太极拳教完，何大夫告诉学员们，光学会太极拳还不够，还要经常练习，最好每天都练习三十分钟，才会对身体健康起作用。如果练习的时候配合呼吸、运气，则效果更好。在最后一次课上，何大夫还邀请到另一位太极专家，两人一起表演了 "太极扇"。两位太极专家动作潇洒大方，刚柔并济，整齐划一。在整个表演过程中，不断有开扇、合扇的 "啪、啪" 声响，既优美悦目，又威武雄壮，把学员们都看呆了。表演结束，掌声雷动。

自从跟何大夫学习太极拳以后，我开始每天早晨练习。在那之前我还学习过气功，所以从 2005 年开始，我晨练的内容就包括 30 分钟气功 + 30 分钟太极拳，几年过去，感觉效果不错，身体不再是 "亚健康" 状态。美国是强调 "生命在于运动" 的国家。2008 年，我所在的明尼苏达大学大力提倡教职员工定期到健身房锻炼身体，并提供种种优惠，包括使用学校的游泳池。我去试游过一个学期以后，又喜欢上了游泳，决定增加游泳这个运动健身项目，而且逐渐加大游泳运动的频率和强度，从每星期两次增加到三次；每次从五十米、一百米、二百米 …… 一直增加到一千多米，而且中间基本不休息。到疫情前，也就是 2018、2019 年时，我感觉身体非常好，比十四、五年前好多了。每年的年度体检，身体的各项指标，包括血压、血脂、血糖、血小板、红、白血球等均在正常范围。因为身体健康，精神状态也非常不错，心情愉快，乐观豁达。我把这些归功于练太极拳、气功和游泳，认为是这几项运动改善了我的健康状况。

2020 年，疫情来袭，为减少病毒传播的风险，学校的健身房关闭了，我也从那年 3 月份开始，被迫停止了游泳健身，到现在已经两年半。加上明州冬季酷寒，室外运动几乎不可能，连跑步都受不了，所以在这几年的冬春季，我几乎没法进行任何室外运动。从那时至今，我的运动健身内容只剩下打太极拳和练气功，而且冬春季只能在室内进行。由于气功的动作很少，所以就"运动"而言，我实际上只有太极拳一项。在运动量大大减少的情况下，那两年多的时间里，我很担心身体状况变差。没想到今年四月份年度体检结果出来，我的各项指标仍然都在正常范围。毫无疑问，这是坚持练太极拳的结果。

出乎意料的是：一个偶然的机会，我还被请上舞台表演太极拳。事情是这样的：2018 年，我所在的明华合唱团在年度演出中，有一个男声小合唱节目"滚滚长江东逝水"。这是明代文学家杨慎的古词"临江仙"，这首词由著名作曲家谷建芬谱曲，作为电视连续剧《三国演义》的片头曲。我们唱的版本有一个将近一分钟的前奏。在这么长的时间里，小合唱的十几个男生在舞台上呆呆地站着，一点动作都没有，演员和观众都会觉得很尴尬。于是在排练时，有团员提出让我在前奏的这一分钟里表演太极拳。刚一听到这个建议，我有点诧异，但转而一想，《三国演义》演绎的是大江东去，浪淘尽，千古风流人物的波澜壮阔、悠久厚重的中国历史，"滚滚长江东逝水"表达的是胸怀上下五千年，古今多少事，都付笑谈中的博大情怀，而太极拳则是数千年中国历史文化积淀的精华，这三者的结合是对中国历史文化的综合表现，可以大大丰富这个节目的内涵。于是我欣然应允。接受任务后，我找明州另一位太极拳高手商量，从何大夫教给我的 24 式简化太极拳中提炼了几个动作，再加上另外几个动作，组合成一套刚柔相济、非常简短的微型太极拳，以"滚滚长江东逝水"的前奏为背景音乐练习。演出那天,男声小合唱的演员们在舞台上站成一排,幕布缓缓拉开,音乐响起。配合动作,我在心里默念:双脚分开与肩同宽,沉肩垂肘,气沉丹田,起势…开始演练这一套微型太极拳。前奏结束,太极拳收势,演唱正好开始。指挥、团员、观众都非常满意,认为前奏时演练的这一段太极拳大大地提高了这个节目的质量,为它加分不少。

作者在《明华合唱团》2018年度演出时表演了太极拳(图15),显然,练太极拳不但让我体质增强,享受健康,还让我把它和艺术结合起来,获得快乐。

52. Becoming A Better Person
成为更好的人

By Zheng Ruolin

I am 59 years old. I have suffered from many diseases, such as allergic rhinitis, bronchitis, nervous headache, etc. What's worse is that my personality has become impatient, angry, and often angry.

In 1974, I had angina pectoris and was diagnosed with coronary heart disease. In addition, I often caught colds and coughed when the weather became cold. After being treated in many large hospitals to little effect, I became very distressed.

In 1977, when I was recuperating, I began to learn Taijiquan from Teacher Sun. After I was discharged from the hospital, I continued to practice Taijiquan. A year later, my bronchitis was cured. Two years later, my neuropathic headache was also completely cured, and the coronary heart disease also improved year by year.

In 1987, I learned Yang Style Taijiquan from Master He Ming, and my Taijiquan skill has made great progress. From 1990 to 1991, I won the Chongqing Taijiquan Exhibition Award for two consecutive years. I am very grateful to my two Taijiquan teachers for their help!

Now, my coronary heart disease symptoms have completely disappeared, I have no more angina pectoris or chest tightness, I catch far fewer colds, and I no longer take medicine every day. In the past, due to my illness, not only was I unable to do housework, but I was also very grumpy, pessimistic, and disappointed. I always felt that life was boring, which made my family worry. Since practicing Taijiquan, I feel that my troubles are gone, and my life is beautiful. I have no worries or anger, and I am full of confidence for the future.

The children say that their mother has changed and has become more cultivated and cheerful. Now I can help with housework, take care of my grandchildren, and become a community Taijiquan instructor. I never imagined that my body could have become healthier as I age, nor that my temper could be tamed with time. The family lives a sweet and beautiful life now, which stems from the happiness that Taijiquan brought me.

I deeply feel that Taijiquan can not only cure diseases, and it makes people better.

我 59 岁了，曾患过许多病，如：过敏性鼻炎，气管炎，神经性头痛等，更糟糕的是性格变的急躁，爱发火，还常常生气。1974 年发生心绞痛，医院确诊患了冠心病，此外还经常感冒，天一冷就咳嗽，经多家大医院治疗，效果不佳，十分苦恼。

1977 年我在疗养时，开始向孙老师学习太极拳，出院后，仍坚持练拳，一年后，气管炎痊愈。两年后神经性头痛也全好了，冠心病亦逐年好转。

1987 年我又拜何明为老师，学习杨式太极拳。拳术有了较大的进步。1990 年至 1991 年，连续两年获重庆市太极拳表演赛优胜奖。我非常感谢两位老师给我的帮助。

现在，我的冠心病症状已经完全消失，再不心绞痛、胸闷了，感冒少多了，也不再经常吃药了。过去因多病，我不仅做不了家务，脾气还很大，悲观失望，总觉得活着没意思，让家里人耽心，自从练拳后，我觉得烦恼没了，生活美好，整天无忧无虑，对未来充满信心，也不再发火了。孩子们都说妈妈变了，越来越有修养，越来越开朗了。现在我能帮助做家务，带孙子，还当了业余武术教练，我万万没想到老来后的身体反比年轻时还健康，老了脾气反而变好了。一家人生活得甜甜美美，这都是太极拳给我带来的幸福。

我深深感到，太极拳既能治病，又能让人变的更好．

53. Bipolar Disorder 躁郁症

Cass Erickson

I have been doing Taijiquan for about six weeks now and the effects of doing it are wonderful and surprising. I took a class with Dr. He last spring and was fascinated by the practice but thought it was probably too complicated for me. But I bought Dr. He's video and thought there may come a time in the future when I'd take the time to learn and practice it. And that time came when I began to have a lot of anxiety. Since western medicine is not an option for me, I popped in the tape one day and gave it a try. Shortly thereafter, I noticed that I was happier and no longer anxious. Now if I miss a day, the anxiety comes back, and I notice that my anxious energy resides in my lungs where I feel a shortness of breath and a fluttering sensation. When I practice Taijiquan, my energy and breath feel evenly distributed throughout my body. I feel balanced and strong. I was delighted to find that Taijiquan can help with bipolar disorder.

I am so happy to notice that Taijiquan is a weight-bearing exercise. Already, my bones feel stronger, and I feel stronger both mentally and physically. Other beneficial effects that I have noticed from Taijiquan are more energy and stamina, improved memory, better balance and coordination, and a general sense of well-being.

I appreciate being given this gift by Dr. He and plan to practice Taijiquan for the rest of my life.

我已经练了太极拳大约六个星期了，效果非常棒和令人惊讶。上个春天我上了何大夫的太极拳课，觉得太难。我买了太极拳带子，准备将来有时间好好学。那段时间我有很多的焦虑，我不想选择用西药，我决定试试太极拳。我开始每天练习太极拳感到开心，如果少做一天太极拳，焦虑就会回来。有时我感到焦虑、能量停留在我的肺部，呼吸短促，身体颤动，练太极拳后就呼吸平稳，身体平静、平衡、有力量，我高兴地发现太极拳可以帮助燥郁症 。现在我感到骨关节有劲，身体强壮，有能量，耐力好，能放松，记忆力提高了，整个身体感到很舒服，有幸福感。

谢谢何大夫给我的礼物，我要一辈子要练太极拳。

54. Get Through Emotionally Difficult Times In The Relationship
度過感情困难时刻

By Julia M. Chavira

I am 38 years old and in my first year of the Masters of Acupuncture program in MN. I had never done Taijiquan before Dr. He's class. At first, I was ambivalent about it; I didn't believe or doubt its abilities to balance, heal, or invigorate, I just thought it was lovely to watch and I hoped I could perform well enough to pass the required class. This sideline view quickly changed as I continued through the 12-week class. I tend to always be chilled with cold limbs and extremities; this was the first change I noticed: I was warm! And the more I did it, the more stable my body temperature became!

Next, I had some major relationship stress going on when class began but with Taijiquan, I felt calmer and more levelheaded during confrontations. A "certain person" can't do Taijiquan and was extremely volatile, but I kept my cool by going into my room and doing 10 minutes of Taijiquan! Often, I would experience headaches, heart palpitations, stomach pain, and distension during these emotionally trying times. No more! Taijiquan is helping with all these issues! I am warmer, calmer, and more centered than I have ever been in my 38 years. Yahoo!

Furthermore, when my 3.5-year-old son is wound up and I don't know what to do with or for him now I just do 10-20 minutes of Taijiquan, and he immediately calms down and mellows out! He copies me or sits quietly; it is amazing!!! I am extremely thankful TCM has found me, and I know the secrets of longevity, balance, health, and inner peace. Taijiquan is phenomenal, life-changing, and well worth learning!

Just think how the world would change if leaders got together and did 20 minutes of Taijiquan first!

Thank you most respectfully, Dr. He!

我今年 38 岁，这是我在明尼苏达州攻读针灸硕士课程的第一年。我以前从来没有练过太极拳。一开始，我对此感到矛盾，我不相信或怀疑它的平衡、治愈或恢复活力的能力。我只是觉得它看起来很有趣，我希望我能表现得足够好，能够通过所要求的课程。随着我继续学习为期 12 周的课程，我的这种观点很快就发生了变化。过去我总是感到很冷，四肢冷。练习太极拳后，我注意到的第一个变化：我变暖和了！我练习得越多，我的体温就越稳定，太棒了！

接下来，太极拳课刚开始时我正面临一些重大的亲属之间的压力。但练习太极拳后，我面对冲突时可以平静、更冷静地去处理。如"某人"不会打太极拳，脾气暴躁，反复无常，我为了保持冷静，便回到自己的房间打 10 分钟太极拳，于是就冷静下来了！我经常在情绪紧张时会有头痛、心悸、胃痛和腹胀，太极拳帮助我解决了所有这些问题。我比 38 年前任何时候都更温暖、更平静、思想更集中。耶！

此外，当我 3 岁半的儿子过于兴奋，我不知道该怎么办，或能为他做什么时，现在我只要做了 10-20 分钟的太极拳，他就立即冷静下来，放松了！他会模仿我，或者静静地坐着；这真是太惊人了！我非常感谢 TCM 中医塑造了我，我知道长寿、平衡、健康和内心平静的秘密。太极拳是非凡的，它能改变生活，非常值得去学习太极拳！

想想看，如果各国领导人聚在一起，先打 20 分钟太极拳，世界将会发生怎样的变化？

非常地感谢您，何医生！

55. To Interact Better with Others
与人交流更好

By Sharon Jeziorski

I have studied with Dr. He since January 2005. Even though I feel I need to learn and practice more, I have seen positive benefits. Since studying Taijiquan, I have noticed people calling or getting into contact with me that I haven't talked to in a while. I also noticed how my students—I am teaching elementary school part-time—have more calm behavior and interactions in general. I also noticed a difference in my balance and flexibility in my ankles during dance class – I study Middle Eastern Dance.

I am very pleased and will continue to study Taijiquan and practice.

我在 2005 年 1 月跟何大夫学太极拳，虽然我还要用更多时间学习与练习，但我已看到正面的好处。自从学太极拳后，与人交流变好。我注意到有一段时间没有联系我的人打电话联系我了。我在小学做兼职，我还注意到我和我的学生—在总体上更融洽和互动。我现正在学跳中东舞，在舞蹈课上，我发现脚踝的平衡和灵活性变好了，

我非常喜欢继续学太极拳，练太极拳。

56. Taijiquan helping control mind
太极拳助守神

By Fangming Xu, Ph.D

There are many benefits to practicing Taijiquan. What I have experienced the most is that Taijiquan helps control the spirits.

Before practicing Taijiquan, as long as I had free time, I would have a lot of thoughts, wild thoughts, crazy thoughts, and I even enjoyed it. But after a long time, the side effects also appeared, manifested in not being able to concentrate when thinking, seriously affecting the study and work, sleep is also affected, and eventually lead to restlessness, in a trance all day long. I wanted to stop thinking, but I couldn't.

When practicing Taijiquan, it is required to relax, remain calm, sink the Qi into the Dantian (in the lower abdomen), and exert with ming, not force. These are extremely helpful in controlling the mind. When I first started practicing Taijiquan, I still had a lot of thoughts and couldn't get into a calm mind. However, with the increase in practice time, I can gradually relax, enter tranquility, and experience the wonderful state of Qi sinking into my Dantian, so that I can keep my mind in Dantian when there is nothing to do. Gradually, my thoughts were also controlled, I stopped thinking wildly, and I slept better. When I feel uneasy, I can immediately focus my mind in Dantian, and I will soon be able to calm down, keep my mind, and prevent it from leaking of mind. Since then, I will no longer be affected by bad emotions such as blind-disordered thinking and anxiety.

Practicing Tai Chi really changed my mood!

练习太极拳有太多的益处，本人体会最深的是太极拳对守神的帮助。

在练习太极拳之前，只要闲下，就会思绪万千，天马行空，胡思乱想，而且，自己也乐此不彼。但时间长了，副作用也显现了，表现在该集中思想时却不能，严重影响了学习和工作，睡眠也受影响，而且最于导致心神不宁，终日处于恍惚状态。自己想停止思绪，却无能为力。

练习太极拳时，要求松、静、气沉丹田、用意不用力，这些对控制心神极有帮助。刚开始练习太极拳时，仍然思绪万千，不能入静。但随着练习时间的增长，慢慢地就能放松了，能入静了，更能体会到气沉丹田的妙境，以致于平时无事之时，都能保持意念守丹田。渐渐地，我的思绪也得到了控制，不再会胡思乱想了，睡眠也好了。遇到心神不安时，立刻意守丹田，很快就能平复心境，守住心神，不让外泄。从此，不再受胡思、焦虑等不良情绪的影响。

练习太极拳真的改变了我的心境！

J   Other Diseases
其它系统疾病

57. A Case of Golden Rooster Standing on One Leg & Deep Breathing Helped a Parkinson's Patient Start Walking
金鸡独立和深呼吸帮助帕金森病人起步走的一例报告

By He Lei

The Japanese patient, male, 70 years old, was first diagnosed in 2013with Parkinson's disease in a general hospital in Yokohama city, and started taking dopamine drugs and using the dopamine receptor agonist patch. The patient's friend introduced him to my clinic for acupuncture and massage treatment. His main complaint was that he had difficulty in starting to walk, and his speech gradually became unclear. Upper limb movements were relatively normal. He comes to the clinic once a week, and every time he suffers from stiffness in his back, shoulders and neck. After receiving the treatment, his body feels relaxed, it becomes easier to start walking, and he can walk more freely on the way home than before. He is very happy about the treatment. For all the patients who come to my clinic for treatment, if necessary, I will teach the self-practice methods to help them recover, mainly come from the guidance technique of Baduanjin and Taijiquan. Of course, the patient needs even more rehabilitation training.

Considering that the difficulty in starting to walk is a problem with moving the center of gravity, I immediately remembered that the center of gravity movement practice of Taijiquan can be used.

So he was advised to start practicing Taijiquan. Speaking of Taijiquan, he said that his wife was practicing, I saidit was just right, wouldn't it be better for a couple to practice! But he looked embarrassed and said he didn't like Taijiquan. I explained: that is good, you can do some of them, of the gravity movement of Taijiquan will help you "start walking". How about you just making a "start"? I show him: take a deep breath and lift hands, exhale and press hands down and bend the knee, then shift your weight to the right foot, and step the left foot to the left (the Wild Horse's Mane on Both Sides in 24-style Taijiquan), just "start"! Teach him to try to do several times, this move is very clever, he can really easily lift the left foot to start away, he was excited, did not expect so simple, so agreed to practice independently, easily lift the left foot to start away.

Seven days later, he came back, and I asked him how effective the practice was. He said it was OK, but it was tootime-consuming. It was some trouble to make a start before doing anything, but taking a deep breath was really good. Later, he gave up Taijiquan, but kept practicing how I taught him breathing. He wrote on his blog: "Repeated two or three deep lead breaths can improve physical activity." And he wrote:" The foundation of my health is the deep breathing of the guide." He called the deep breath I taught him" deep guide, "and the difference from the" x-style deep breath" I did before, he summed up at least three points: 1. When inhaling, close the abdomen without expanding it; 2. Exhale. When breathing, close your mouth and use your nose instead of exhaling through your mouth; 3.keep your head and body upright, and look ahead. He mentioned in his blog his interest in ancient Chinese "immortals", which was one of his motivation for his practice.

Although abandoning Taijiquan, the deep breathing method from Taijiquan did help him. Every time he went to the hospital, the doctor asked him to walk to see if his gait had deteriorated. He drove the "deep breath" to show a natural start, and the doctor was surprised to twist his neck: how could this man's disease progress so slowly (he complacently reported to me).

Four years later, the doctor wondered if the diagnosis was wrong, so he did the tests again, including MIBG scan and DAT scan, confirmed that he was undoubtedly Parkinson's disease, and continued dopa medicine treatment.

Five years later, his illness progressed little by little. He was still not enthusiastic about Taijiquan practice, his speech was gradually unclear, and he felt more and more difficult to move in the relatively narrow environment at home. The hospital introduced him to start rehabilitation training." Start to walk" training is a very common practice: crossing obstacles. PT is very enthusiastic, and he is very carefully trained to cross obstacles to help to start, but not everywhere there are available obstacles in front of his feet, so he invented the English letter "L" crutch: a stick parallel to the ground to the bottom end of the ordinary crutch. The usage is to put the L-shaped walking stick in front of the foot, staring down at the horizontal stick in front of the foot, and step over . Although it is possible to start walking, the horizontal bar hinders walking. Focusing on the bar in front of his feet, he forgot to take deep breaths, and the biggest drawback is to affect his posture: looking down at the bar in front of his feet, making him more like a Parkinson's posture!

His condition prompted me to help him find a simpler way to "start". At this time, his starting foot twitched several times in place, making it difficult to take a step.. And his hands also move freely, yes, can use his hands to drive the feet, help the center of gravity move! There are many scenes where the hands and feet of Taijiquan move at the same time, which can be used. "Golden Rooster Independence" comes to my mind.

The "downward potential independence" of Type 24 Taijiquan is my favorite potential. For this patient who does not like to practice Taijiquan, I had to first omit the "inferior potential" and directly do the "independence". Lift the same side of the hands and feet together, -with the hand to drive the feet, wonderful cooperation-is appropriate. And compared with the "starting" side walk, the golden rooster can move forward independently, which is more conducive to starting and walking forward!

He already has the right way to breathe. I instructed him to lift the hands and feet on the same side forcefully while inhaling, so that he could instantly shift the center of gravity to the supporting feet, and the feet that were lifted during the instability landed, just enough to start walking!

It worked, which he learned at once. But sometimes only the hand are raised, and the foot can not be raised. When this situation appears, I guide him: first pat the same side of the thigh with the hand, concentrate on directing the "qi" to the leg that you want to move, then exhale and bend both knees slightly at the same time, then While inhaling, lift up the same side of the hand and foot with one breath;try doing this for 1 or 2 times, then you can lift your foot and start walking. Parkinson's disease is an intractable disease. I have initially observed that the "deep breathing" exercise can delay the progression of the disease. The "Golden Rooster Independence" can help patients quickly "start to walk". Regular practice of the "Golden Rooster Independence" can also help maintain a sense of balance. There may be clues to solving Parkinson's disease, which are worthy of further study. This is my expectation

I always wonder, if my patient liked to practice Taijiquan, would it be more effective? Anyway, Taijiquan helped him, and this example might help more Parkinson's patients. Don't forget to let me know if your practice comes to fruition. The author is engaged in clinical work of acupuncture and massage in his acupuncture clinic in Yokohama, Japan. His email: drhelei@yahoo.co.jp

患者日本人，男性，70 岁，2013 年初诊。在横滨市某综合医院诊断为帕金森病，开始服用多巴胺类药物及使用多巴胺受体激动剂贴剂。经病人的友人介绍来我的诊所接受针灸按摩治疗。他的主诉是，起步走困难，渐渐语言不清，上肢活动比较正常。每周来诊一次，每次都是背部及肩颈僵硬，接受治疗后会感觉身体轻松，起步走变得容易，回家的路途也比来时行走自如，他很高兴。

来我诊所接受治疗的所有病人，如果有必要我都会教授帮助他们康复的自我练习方法，这些方法主要来自于以八段锦为主的导引术和太极拳等。这个病人当然更是需要康复训练。

考虑到起步走困难是在重心移动上有问题，我立即想起太极拳的重心移动练习可以利用，所以建议他开始练习太极拳。说起太极拳，他说其夫人在练习，我说正好啊，夫妇练习不是更好嘛！但他一脸难色，说自己不喜欢太极拳。我解释说：那好，不全部做也可以，太极拳的重心移动，对你"起步走"会有帮助。要不然，你就只做一个"起势"怎么样？我做给他看：深吸气抬双手，呼气下按双手并曲膝，接着重心移动到右脚上，向左迈出左脚（24 式太极拳的野马分鬃），正好"起步走"！教给他试着做了几次，这招很灵，他果然可以轻松的抬起左脚起步走了，他兴奋起来，没想到这么简单，于是同意自主练习，轻松的抬起左脚起步走，回家去了。

7 天后他来复诊，我问他练习的效果如何，他说还好，就是太费时间，做什么事之前都要做一个起势有些麻烦，但深呼吸确实不错。后来，他放弃了太极拳，但一直练习我教给他呼吸法。他在自己的 blog 写道："重复做 2 ～ 3 次导引术的深呼吸后，可以改善身体活动。"并且写着："我的健康的基本，在于导引术的深呼吸。"

他称我教给他的深呼吸为"导引术的深呼吸"，与遇到我之前做的"x式的深呼吸"的区别，他总结至少有三点：1，吸气时收腹而不鼓腹部；2，呼气时闭口用鼻，而不是用口呼气；3，保持头和身体正直，目视前方。他在自己的 blog 中提到他对中国古代的"神仙术"颇有兴趣，这也是他坚持练习的动机之一。

虽然放弃了太极拳，但从太极拳开始的深呼吸方法确实帮助了他。每去医院复诊，医生会让他走一走，看看他的步态是否恶化。他都会使用"导引术的深呼吸"来展示比较自然的起步走，医生每次都会吃惊不解拧转脖子：这个人病情怎么会如此进展缓慢（他自满的向我报告）。

四年过去，医生觉得奇怪，是不是诊断错误了，于是又检查，包括 MIBG scan 和 DAT scan，确诊他无疑是帕金森病，继续多巴类药物治疗。五年过去了，他的病情一点点进展，他对太极拳的练习依然没有热度，说话渐渐不清楚，感到在家里比较狭窄的环境里移动也越来越困难了，医院介绍他开始康复训练。"起步走"的训练是很普通的做法：即跨越障碍物。西医的 PT 很热心，他也很认真接受训练，跨越障碍物确实有助于起步，但不是任何地方都刚好脚前有可利用的障碍物，无奈之下，他竟自己发明了英文字母"L"字形的拐杖：即在普通拐杖的最下端连接一个与地面平行的棒。用法是把 L 字拐杖放在脚前，低头眼盯着脚前的横棒，跨越过去。虽然可以起步走，但横棒却妨碍步行。由于专注于脚前的横棒，竟然忘记了深呼吸，而且最大的缺点是影响姿势：低头看脚前的横棒，让他更像帕金森姿态！

他的状况促使我帮助他找到更简捷的"起步走"方法。这时他起步的脚在原地抽搐几次，难以迈出步子。而他的手还活动自如，对，可以用手带动脚，帮助重心移动！太极拳手脚同时动作的场面比比皆是，可以利用。我想到了"金鸡独立"。

24 式太极拳的"下势独立"是我喜欢的势子，对于这个不爱练习太极拳的病人，只好先省略"下势"直接做"独立"了。同侧的手脚一起抬起，—用手带动脚，绝妙的配合—正合适。而且与"起势"的侧方走相比，金鸡独立可以向前迈步，更有利于向前方起步行走！

他已经有了正确的呼吸方法的基础。我指导他在吸气的同时用力抬同侧的手脚，这样可以一瞬间把重心移动到支撑脚上，在不稳中抬起的脚落地，刚好可以起步走！

这一招可行，他马上就学会了。但有时会只有手抬起来，而脚抬不起来的现象。这种情况出现时，我指导他：先用手拍拍同侧的大腿前侧，集中精力也就是把"气"引导到想要动的腿上，随后呼气并且同时稍微曲两膝，然后吸气的同时"一气"抬起同侧手足，这样试做 1 ～ 2 次，即可以抬起脚起步走了。

帕金森病是难治疾病，我初步观察到了"导引术的深呼吸"练习可以延缓病情恶化的进程，金鸡独立可以帮助病人快捷"起步走"，经常练习金鸡独立的动作，还可以帮助维持平衡感觉。其中也许隐藏着解决帕金森病的线索，值得深入研究。这是我的期待。

我总是在想，如果我的这位病人喜欢练习太极拳，结果是不是效果会更理想一些呢？无论如何，太极拳帮助了他，这个例子也许会帮助更多的帕金森患者。如果练习有了结果，别忘了告诉我一声。

作者在日本横浜市的针灸诊所从事针灸推拿的临床工作。
email：drhelei@yahoo.co.jp

58. Mononucleosis 单核细胞增多症

By Alexandria Rice

In the past seven to eight months, I have developed a disease called Mononucleosis. It made me feel particularly tired, with headaches, and a sore throat. I stayed in bed for about three months back then, and I began to regain energy during the fourth month. But having spent that long a period doing little more than sleeping and eating, I physically became very weak, and even walking up a flight of stairs was difficult – this was partially due to the virus itself, but my muscles were significantly weaker as well. Also, it was difficult for me to process things mentally as I has not been using my mind much during this time, and I also had a continuous headache. Emotionally everything was very difficult for me to take in and deal with. Everything in life seemed HUGE and I wanted to hide away from most problems.

As I said, about 4 months after I acquired mono, I began to regain some energy, though it was a slow process, and I began some schoolwork again and tried to take slow, short walks outside. About a month later (around the fifth month of my illness) I began a Taijiquan class, hoping to regain some strength and get some exercise. Also, the Traditional Chinese Medicine Doctor I had been seeing suggested that I begin to exercise more. I thought it would help physically, but I didn't really think about the mental or emotional effects it could have.

I had a class once a week and I practiced an average of six days a week. I usually practiced from 15 to 30 minutes a day. I know I have a lot more to learn and that when I am more practiced at Taijiquan I will probably be affected more by it, but it has already helped me to heal and grow in the past three months. I am much stronger than I was. I can practice for 30 minutes now (sometimes more) before I start to shake (whereas in the beginning, I was shaking the whole time I practiced). Also, I can concentrate on schoolwork for longer periods of time. Emotionally I have been affected as well, and I believe it was partially Taijiquan that contributed to that. I am a lot more responsive, rather than reactive. I pause to think about my decisions in life along with what I say to others. I really try not just react to life and those around me.

I do not know how remarkable my experience with Taijiquan is to others. But for me, it has given shape and new energy to my life. I plan on doing Taijiquan for the rest of my days.

在过去的 7 到 8 个月里，我得了一种病，西医称作"单核白血球增多症"。它使我感到特别的累，头痛，喉咙痛。那时我在床上呆了大约三个月，在第四个月才恢复精神，但是在这么长的时间里只有睡觉和吃饭，我的身体在变弱，连上几步楼梯都很难，这是病毒对我的影响，我的肌肉也明显地变弱了。我很难处理事情，因为在这段时间我没有使用过我的头脑，我一直头痛。不管什么事情对我来说都是非常困难去参与或处理。生活中的一切看起来那么复杂，我想躲避。

在第四个月，我开始恢复一些能量，它是一个缓慢的过程，我开始做点功课了，我试图慢慢的走路。大约一个月后（應該是在第五个月），我开始参加太极拳班，希望能恢复一些力量，得到一些锻炼。我的中医师也叫我要多锻炼一点。我认为这将有助於我的身体，但我没多想太极拳对於我精神和情绪上会有产生什么样的影响。

我每周上一次课，平均每周练习 6 天。我通常每天练习 15 到 30 分钟。我知道我还有很多东西要学，当我更多地练习太极拳时，我可能会受到更多的影响，但在过去的三个月里，太极拳已经帮助我愈合和成长。我比以前强壮多了，我现在可以练习 30 分钟 (有时更多)，然后才开始力不从心 (而在开始的时候，我在整个练习的时间里都在摇晃)。而且，我可以花更长的时间专心学习。情感上我也受到了影响，我可以更长时间地专注于学校的工作。我相信是太极拳部分地促成了这一点，我的反应更灵敏，而不是被动的。我可以停下来思考我在生活中的决定以及我对别人说的话，我真的试着不只是对生活和我周围的人做出被动反应。

　　我不知道我的太极拳经验对别人来说有多了不起。但对我来说，它塑造了我的生活，给了我新的能量。我打算余生都打太极拳。

59. Renal Insufficiency 肾功能不全

By Margaret Nordeen

I saw Dr. He in the summer of 2016 because I was experiencing lower back pain, fatigue and stiffness in my right hip (I had just broken my right hip in Feb. and was recovering from hip-replacement surgery).

In addition, by 2016, I had suffered from diabetes for 52 years (diagnosed as a child) and was concerned about developing kidney complications. Back in 2016, my Creatinine serum level was elevated - Cr 1.01 (On a range between 0.50-0.9). Dr. He recommended Taijiquan daily to improve kidney function.

I have continued to do the 24-Form Taijiquan for the past six years, three or four times a week. Not only have my Creatinine numbers decreased to 0.89 but overall, Taijiquan has benefited me with better control of diabetes, improved circulation, and lower blood sugar. Deep breathing helps my cardio-respiratory function, improves my balance, decreases stress, and improved my flexibility.

I feel healthier today than I have for decades. Taijiquan is gentle and can be done anywhere and it will continue to be part of my self-care regimen.

2016年夏天，我开始看何医生。因为我的右髋关节感到疲劳和僵硬，还有腰痛.（2月时我的右髋关节刚刚骨折，正在从髋关节置换手术中恢复）。

此外，到2016年，我患糖尿病已经52年（小时候被诊断I型糖尿病），很担心会出现肾脏并发症。在 2016 年，我的肾功能血清肌酐水平就升高到 Cr 1.01（正常是 0.50-0.99）。何医生建议每天练习太极拳来改善肾功能。

在过去的六年里，我坚持练习 24 式太极拳，每周做三到四次。太极拳不仅让我的肌酐水平降低到 0.89，而且让我能更好地控制糖尿病，还改善血液循环，降低血糖。深呼吸则有助于心脏呼吸功能，更好的平衡身体，减少压力和提高身体的灵活性。

我现在的感觉比几十年来都更健康。太极拳是温和的，可以在任何地方做，它将继续是自我护理方案的一部分。

60. Anemia and Rheumatic Heart Disease
贫血和风湿性心脏病

By Wu YingFang

In 1960, I suffered from severe iron deficiency anemia. I often passed out. After only two years of high school, I dropped out of high school. In 1972, I was diagnosed with severe rheumatic heart disease with mitral valve stenosis. My ESR was 85mm/hour, with lower extremity edema. The temperature in Chongqing was as often as high as 39 degrees Celsius, yet I had to wear a sweater. I was so skinny that I was bedridden all day because of fatigue, palpitation, and difficulty breathing. I looked for magical doctors everywhere and exhausted all the panaceas in China, but the disease was still not cured. I struggled for my life and felt that there was no way out.

In 1974, my children helped me go to the park to learn Taijiquan from Master He Ming. I diligently practiced Yang-style Taijiquan, Taijiquan sword, Taijiquan knife, and I did not even rest on Sundays. After the first month of practice, my body was sore, and I couldn't get up from squatting. After practicing Taijiquan for 8 months, my body was much better. My house was only one stop away from the park. In the past, with the support of my children, I had to rest many times before arriving. Now I can walk easily by myself, my ESR has dropped to 15mm/hour, the hemoglobin is normal, I don't need to wear sweaters in summer anymore, and I no longer have heart palpitations. Since 1975, my sick leave has been largely eliminated. My companion surprisingly asked me "How did you cure your illness?" I said, "I was cured by Master He Ming in the Park. The Yang-style Taijiquan he taught me is more effective than medicine."

I was able to go from a patient with severe anemia and rheumatic heart disease to a healthy community Taijiquan instructor, all thanks to Taijiquan.

1960年我因患严重缺铁性贫血，经常昏倒，高中只读了两年就休学了。1972年经医院确诊患了严重的风湿性心脏病；二尖瓣狭窄。血沉85mm/小时，下肢浮肿。重庆热天温度高达39度，我还得穿毛衣。人瘦得皮包骨头。因疲乏，心慌，呼吸困难，整天卧床不起。我到处求医看病吃药，病还是医不好。真是："久病四处求神医，灵丹妙药都吃尽。就是不能治我病，苦与死神把命争"，我真感到走头无路。

1974年孩子们扶我去公园向何明老师学太极拳，星期天也不休息。我学会了杨氏太极拳，剑，刀。第一月练下来。全身酸疼，蹲着就起不来了。8个月后身体就好多了。我家去公园只一站路，过去在孩子的扶持下还要休息好多次才能走到。现在自己一人轻轻松松地就走到了，血沉已经下降到15mm/小时了，血色素也正常了，夏天也不用再穿毛衣了，心也不慌了。从1975年起基本不再请病假了。同伴惊奇地问我："你的病在哪儿医好的？"我说："我是在沙坪公园何明老师那里治好的，他教我的杨氏太极拳比药还管用呢"。

我能从一个严重的贫血病，风湿性心脏病患者，变成身体健康的业余武术教练，这都是打太极拳的功劳．

K   The Little Experience of Practicing Taijiqua 练太极拳的点滴体会

61. The Benefit of Taijiquan 太极拳的好处

Wen Hong， You Benzhong professor 教授

Taijiquan practice is a great experience for us under Dr. He's excellent teaching!

All the different forms engage our body & mind, strengthening our muscles & ability to balance!

It uplifts our spirit & helps us stay calm in the face of challenges in life!

We shall make Taijiquan a part of our life!

在何博士的指导下练习太极拳是一次非常棒的经历！

所有不同的形式都让我们的身心参与进来，加强我们的肌肉和平衡能力！它能振奋我们的精神，帮助我们在面对生活中的挑战时保持冷静！

我们要让太极拳成为我们生活的一部分！

62. Taijiquan Brought Me Prestige
太极拳让我获得威望

By Virginia Wood

I am a special education teacher working at Hiawatha Elementary School. My responsibilities also include standing in the West Corridor and managing students coming and going to school. Unfortunately, many students run around and don't listen to me. Because I am neither the principal nor an academic teacher, the students sometimes don't respect me as a chaperone. So many times, my efforts to maintain order were futile and the students ignored me completely.

This autumn, nature gave us a pleasant surprise. I took advantage of the beautiful weather to practice Taijiquan during my lunch break. I didn't notice that the place where I practiced was visible from the student cafeteria. The principal asked me to be careful not to practice Taijiquan in front of the students because it had caused a commotion among the dining students.

I followed her instructions but soon noticed that the students started to obey me very consciously. Apparently, they saw me practicing Taijiquan and thought I was a martial arts master.

As a result, I have gained high prestige among my students, and I no longer need to repeat myself to my students.

我是一位 Hiawatha 小学的特殊教育老师。我的责任还包括站在西边走廊管理上下学时来往的学生。不幸的是我的学生不听我的管教，他们四处乱走乱跑，他们认为我不是校长，不是导师，认为我没有管束他们的权力。因此许多时候，我所做的努力维持秩序都是徒劳无益的，学生们完全无视于我。

这个秋天大自然赠与了我们小阳春，我打算利用这美好的天气在午餐休息时来打太极拳。我没有注意到我练习的地方从学生餐厅里是可以看见的。校长要我注意不要在学生面前练习太极拳，因为已经引起了就餐学生的骚动。

我听从了她的指示。但很快注意到：学生们开始非常自觉地服从于我，显然他们看到了我练太极拳，认为我是武术大师，会功夫。

由此我在学生中获得极高的威望，从此后我再也不需要对学生重复管束的话了。

63. Improved my Balance a Lot
提高了我的平衡能力

By Victor Wang

I have been taking Taijiquan lessons from Steven Yang for the last few months.

He is very enthusiastic about Taijiquan both for himself and as a teacher. Taijiquan is recommended for health reasons, both physical and mental. For senior citizens, it is very helpful for mobility, balance, and coordination. It helps calm down the mind and I prefer it over meditation alone.

Yang takes time to explain every step and is very patient, making sure students understand the proper steps with breathing. I will continue to take lessons from him which have already improved my balance by a lot. He is the kind of person we need in the community, especially when he volunteers his time and knowledge.

在过去的几个月里，我一直在跟 Steven Yang 学习太极拳。

他对太极非常热情，无论是对他自己还是作为一名老师。太极拳是出于身体和心理健康的考虑而被推荐的。对于老年人来说，它对灵活性、平衡和协调都很有帮助。它有助于冷静的头脑，我喜欢它而不是单独冥想。

Steven 花时间讲解每一个步骤，并且非常耐心，确保学生理解呼吸的正确步骤。我将继续向他学习，他已经使我的平衡能力提高了很多。他是我们社区需要的那种人，尤其是当他自愿献出自己的时间和知识的时候。

64. Taiji Has Been One Threshold to Freedom and Timelessness
太极拳是通向自由和永恒的门槛

By Amanda Degener

Early years have a huge impact on how you go through life. I grew up in the inner city of St. Louis in the 1960's where there were gangs and drugs. I had three brothers and we all dealt with it differently. The brother closest to my age had guns. but I just got tough. You had to walk down the street a certain way or you would get messed with. I learned that being sensitive meant getting shoved off your bike and never seeing it again. It seemed dangerous to be soft.

Growing up in the inner city of St. Louis I had to pretend to be tough. If you did not walk down the street a certain way, you would get messed with. It was dangerous to be soft.

It was not until I started playing Taijiquan in 2008 that I found strength in softness. I signed up because I wanted to slow down. Some people need to rev up so maybe they take Zumba classes, but I needed to move at a slower speed. I noticed in the beginner-level classes students often exhausted their patience and gave up, but I stuck with it. As I progressed out of the beginner-level classes my tough crust dissolved and a profound transformation occurred.

Now when I play Taijiquan my body does the thinking, and it's a form of meditation. Taijiquan has helped me to remember that time is not as the 21st century seems to demand. The chaotic world may be speeding by, ever faster and ever-changing, but our needs have not changed. Reflection, nearness, care, and love are found in slowness. Slowness is where we are renewed, where we sense ourselves in the world and find the boundaries of our own existence.

This "doing" seems to include undoing. When playing Taijiquan, the incessant banter of the brain is gone or no longer dominates. The busy body quiets the brain; it brings the mind to a calmer state. This slowness has been one threshold to freedom and timelessness. Slowness is where we are renewed, and where we sense ourselves in the world, where we can explore the boundaries of our existence. There is a restfulness in working with the form till things are fully resolved.

Since I began my daily practice, I am more focused and relaxed. I like to say I am more flexible in my mind and body. Professional athletes, military leaders, businessmen, and the medical profession have already praised both the physical and psychological health advantages of Taijiquan. At 64, I take no prescription medications and I have had no surgeries. I am confident there are many health problems.

I take a little time each morning to give myself the gift of Taijiquan.

早年对一个人的人生有很大的影响。20世纪60年代，我在圣路易斯市中心长大，那里有黑帮和毒品。我有三个兄弟，我们的处理方式都不一样。和我年龄相仿的兄弟都拿起了枪，而我却变得强硬起来。你必须以特定的方式强硬走在街上，否则你会被耍。我明白软弱意味着被人从自行车上推下去，软弱似乎是危险的。我不得不假装坚强。

直到2008年我开始打太极拳，我才在柔软中找到力量。我报名是因为我想慢下来。有些人需要加快速度，所以他们可能会去学桑巴舞，但我需要以较慢的速度移动。我注意到，在初级阶段的课程中，学生们经常耗尽他们的耐心而放弃，但我坚持了下来。当我走出初级课程的时候，我粗暴的性格改变了，即一种深刻的转变发生了。

现在当我打太极拳时，我的身体在思考，这是一种冥想。太极拳让我意识到，时间似乎并不是像 21 世纪所要求的那样，混乱的世界可能正在飞速流逝，速度越来越快，变化越来越多，但我们的需求没有改变。反思、亲近、关心和爱都是在缓慢中发现的，是我们在世界上感知自己并找到自己存在的边界的地方。

在打太极拳时，大脑中不断的玩笑会消失或不再占主导地位。忙碌的身体让大脑安静；它能使人的思想达到一种平静的状态。这种缓慢是通向自由和永恒的一个门槛。缓慢是我们更新的地方，是我们在世界上感知自己的地方，是我们探索我们存在的边界的地方。练习太极拳会让人感到宁静。

自从开始我的日常练习太极拳，我更专注和放松。我喜欢我的身心更加灵活。职业运动员、军事领导人、商人和医学界都对太极拳的身心健康优势赞不绝口。64 岁时，我没有服用过处方药，也没有做过手术。我相信我正在避免许多影响健康的麻烦问题。

我每天早上都会花一点时间打太极拳，作为给自己的礼物。

65. keeping Me in the Present Moment.
活在当下

By Brian Yauk

I have been taking a Taijiquan class hosted by Steven Yang.

Steven has a strong passion for Taijiquan, both for its health benefits and mental discipline. He also is fascinated with studying the underlying scientific principles of why it is beneficial, such as how muscles work or the effects of breathing. He also has a strong passion for sharing his knowledge and experience with others for the benefit of improving people's physical, mental and spiritual health, which can be seen in the excitement he has for teaching it.

Taijiquan has benefitted me by bringing more intention into my breathing, keeping me in the present moment. It has also improved my coordination in the way that I make slow and deliberate movements as part of Taijiquan. Practicing Taijiquan is also a nice way for me to relax and let go of all the events that have happened that day and be present with myself.

我一直在上史蒂文·阳主持的太极拳课。

史蒂文对太极拳有强烈的爱好，因为它对健康有好处，对精神有训练。他还着迷于研究为什么它有益健康的基本科学原理，如肌肉如何工作或呼吸的影响。他也有强烈的热情与他人分享他的知识和经验，以改善人们的身体、心理和精神健康，这可以从他对教授这些知识和经验的兴奋中看出。

太极拳让我的呼吸更有目的性，让我活在当下。它还提高了我的协调能力，使我可以缓慢而从容地做动作，作为太极拳的一部分。练习太极拳对我来说也是一种很好的放松方式，让我放下当天发生的所有事情，太极拳是给我自己的礼物。

66. The Offensive and Defensive Effects of Taijiquan 太极拳的攻防作用

By Simon Fan

In my younger days, I served in the military for few years. Taekwondo was part of the training. I practiced it even after the service. Tai-Chi was just a name until I met Master He. He was a kind and patient man. However, to me, Taijiquan was like a slow exercise and no fighting spirit at all. I was young and I was a person with short-fused temperament (I thought that I was a nice guy but, my wife has different opinion.)

One day after class, I ask a question to Master He. It was simply: How to apply Taijiquan in a hand-to-hand combat (he knew that I was a soldier with some Taekwondo experience). His answer was also simple: keep practiceTaijiquan and you might understand more, later. And, that was not the answer I was looking for. But I kept pushing him my questions and the master kept ignored me, of course.

Another few months passed, the master finally shared two thoughts with me.

Number one: " Push Hands" (推手). I just need to understand its movement.Both hands/arms can move not only from left to right, right to left, but also, up and down, diagonally, front to back, or any direction as your body stance moves (or not moving). When hands are moving, one (in front position) do the blocking and the other follows with attacks (palm or fist), at same time. I applied the "Cloud Hands" with my Taekwondo,

I was surprised how powerful and useful this one little movement can be. Then, I realized that why so many martial arts applied Taijiquan in their technics. I was so happy till these days.

Number two:if you have a quick temperament, learn to control it. Master He knew me well.

Overall, I just want say: how little I know Taijiquan, and, express my appreciation to Master He for his patient with me. His friendly smile is a great reminder for the two thoughts he thought me⋯ especially the number two, of course.

在我年轻的时候，我在军队服役了几年。跆拳道曾经是训练的一部分。在服务之后，我也会练习。太极，在我遇到何明师傅之前，只是一个名词。对我来说，太极拳就像是一种缓慢的运动，完全没有战斗力。何明师傅，是一个善良而有耐心的人。当时，我年轻是个脾气暴躁的人（我认为我是个心地善良的人，但我老婆可能有不同的意见。）

一天下课，我问何老师一个问题。很简单：如何在肉搏战中运用太极拳（他知道我曾是有一点跆拳道经验的人）。他的回答也很简单：继续练太极，以后你可能会明白。但是，这不是我要找的答案。之后，我一直向他提出我的问题，当然，师傅也一直只有微笑，也不理我。又过了几个月，师傅於于与我分享了他的看法。

第一："推手"。要我了解它的动作。双手 / 手臂，不仅可以从左到右、从右到左移动，还可以利用身体姿势移动（或不移动），上下、左右对角斜线、从前到后或任何方向移动。 在移动双手时，一挡，一攻（手掌或拳头），可以同时进行。我把这个动作和我的跆拳道混合在一起，我很惊讶这个小动作，有那么强大和有用。后来，才明白，为什么这么多武术都有太极拳基本动作在里面。直到今天，我都很高兴知道这种格斗技巧。

第二：不要生气。如果你的性情急躁，学会控制它。我只能说，何师傅很了解我我也想说两件事情：第一：对太极拳，知道的太少，太少。第二：感謝何师傅对我的耐心。我永遠記得，何师傅的微笑。微笑，是对我的一个提醒…，尤其是第二个，不要生气。

67. Find the Middle Path 找到中间道路

By Amy Reede

I have practiced Taijiquan for over ten years, and it has been a steady, calming, and strengthening force in my life.

I was inspired to begin school for TCM by Cheng Man-ch'ing (Manqing Zheng), who was a great doctor and teacher of Taijiquan. My first teacher helped me build a good foundation, and led me through breathing exercises and focusing on keeping the energy rooted in my feet - which has helped me maintain balance and rooted in my daily life. With regular practice, I have more energy to accomplish my work and studying as well as prevent or recover faster from illness.

As the qi moves through me, I sometimes feel like I am in a new dimension—very peaceful and calm, yet thinking with clarity.

My teacher said Taijiquan is also called Supreme Ultimate Boxing. —It helps balance yin and yang, so eventually, the body and mind can find the middle way —no deficiency, no excess，Just good！

我练太极拳超过十年，太极拳在我生命中是一个稳定、平和，又使我强壮的力量。

我的第一个太极拳老师给我打了很好的根基。他是程曼清老师，他给了我启发，他是一位优秀的医生、太极拳老师。他引导我做呼吸运动和专注于保持能量根植于脚—这帮助我保持平衡，根植于我的日常生活。有了规律的练习，我有更多的精力来完成我的工作和学习，太极拳帮助我预防和治愈疾病。

当气流过我身体时，我觉得我在一个新的维度——非常平静，思考清晰。

　　我的太极拳老师说这是最高级的拳术，它帮助阴阳平衡，所以终于找到身心平衡，不偏不倚，刚刚好！

68. Taijiquan Has Been an Excellent Exercise 太极拳是一种极好的运动

By John Cowles

As I approach my 80th birthday, I believe that learning the short form has been an excellent exercise for both my brain and my legs and my sense of balance. Aging, I believe, tends to impair one's sense of and ability to maintain balance. The slow shifting of weight from one leg to the other, plus the "Golden Rooster" and the kicks, fully engages the eye and inner ear as well as the muscles of the feet. And the authenticity – the beauty – of the moves when well-executed is felt, even more, I believe, by the performer than by the observer.

It has been a joy to study the beginning of *Taijiquan*.

当我步入我 80 岁的生日时，我相信学短式（24 式）太极拳对我的脑子，腿和平衡是很好的锻炼。我相信老化往往会损害人的意识和能力、平衡。练太极拳缓慢地由一只脚到另一只的转移重心，加上"金鸡独立"和踢腿，训练了眼和内耳以及腿的肌肉。而它真实—美丽的动作，我相信，当太极拳动作完成得很好时，表演者比观看者的感触更多。

学习太极拳是一种乐趣。

69. Learn Taijiquan Makes My balance Improved
学太极拳使我的平衡能力有所改善

By Melinda Spike

This is my first experience with *Taijiquan*. I found the routine to be both fascinating and challenging. My personal goal was just to try to get each move into my muscle memory. This I now know will be a goal to perfect over many years. The gentle motions of this activity will help condition and care for my body for the rest of my life. My balance has improved and is helping me improve my skills in other sports I enjoy. When I leave class, I feel calmer and refreshed.

这是我第一次学太极拳。我发现这些动作既迷人又充满挑战，我个人的目标只是试图让我的肌肉记住每个动作，现在我所学到的将会是我未来完美的目标。这个运动的柔和动作将有助于我和照顾我的身体一辈子。我的平衡能力已有所改善，并帮助我提高我喜欢的其它运动技能。当我上完课后，我觉得更平静和精神焕发。

70. Doing Taijiquan for 20 Minutes Is equal to One Hour Exercise
练太极拳 20 分钟等于其它运动一小时

By Marnie Leen

Practicing 20 minutes of Taijiquan is equivalent to One hour of other exercises.

There are several immediate effects that I have noticed practicing *Taijiquan*. The first is that when I finish the routine in its entirety, there is a surge of energy. It's almost like I have the same sort of endorphin rush that I feel after an hour's of workout at the gym.

The second major effect I have noticed is stress release. Sometimes when my mind is racing, I close my eyes and visualize myself going through the entire routine. By the end of the visualization, I am extremely relaxed and most of the time I have completely forgotten what I had been thinking about.

练习 20 分钟的太极拳相当于一个小时的其他练习。

练太极拳后有几个立竿见影的效果：首先当我练 20 分钟后，就会有一股能量激增，它相当于在运动中心练一小时产生的内啡肽一样。

第二个主要影响是压力的释放。有时我心里烦时，我会闭上眼想象练太极拳的那些动作，想象完之后非常放松，也忘记了许多烦恼事。

71.Stress Level is Significantly Lower
压力明显减轻

By Lisa Smyth

Since I started *Taijiquan* 12 weeks ago, I have found it has not only helped my physical well-being but has also helped clear my mind.

After doing *Taijiquan* my stress level is significantly lower, my concentration is heightened, and my emotional state is joyful.

I suffer from allergies, menstrual problems, and some slight depression from light deficiency. After doing *Taijiquan*, I don't notice these ailments as much.

I recommend *Taijiquan* to anyone who wants to boost his or her immune system, increase energy, and reduce stress.

自从 12 周前我开始练太极拳，我发现它不仅帮助我的健康，也帮助我头脑清晰。

做完太极拳后，我的压力的程度明显偏低，我的注意力提高，我的情绪是快乐的。

我患有过敏症，月经问题和因缺乏光照引起些轻微的抑郁症。练习太极拳之后，我已经不注意到这些毛病了。

我推荐太极拳给任何想要提升免疫力，增强体力和减轻压力的人们。

72. Taijiquan Calms My Mind and Helps Me Sleep
太极拳使我心情平静并帮助我睡眠

By Auchea Sulluian

Taijiquan warms my body. It increases my energy, calms my mind, and helps me sleep. It makes me more aware of my posture weaknesses, Creates a sense of calm focus with graceful action. It helps me become efficient in everyday work.

太极拳温暖了我的身体。增加我的能量，平静了我的心灵，并帮助我入睡。还让我知道到自己的姿势缺点，用优雅的动作创造一种平静的专注感，帮助我在日常工作中变得高效。

73. Taijiquan Makes Me Have a Peaceful Mind. 太极拳使我拥有平和的心态

By Grace Chao

After practicing for 2 months, I feel comfortable when I wake up in the morning. *Taijiquan* practice has increased my blood circulation. It also helps me to be relaxed and refreshed after working a long day.

The most important thing is to remember the proverb from Dr. He – have a peaceful mind.

练习太极拳 2 个月后，我早上醒来时感觉很舒服，增加了血液循环，它还有助于工作一整天后的放松和恢复。

最重要的是记住了何大夫的格言 — 拥有一个平和的心态。

74. Taijiquan Helps My Hip Pain
太极拳缓解了我的髋关节痛

By Manan Abdel-Rahman

I began practicing Taijiquan in January 2005 with Dr. He. I love to practice in my driveway very early in the morning (in a wooded rural area). It helps me feel very alive and happy to be alive. I have trouble with my hips and made an appointment for acupuncture on a Thursday. That Wednesday evening, I practiced Taji in class and had no pain on Thursday.

I think Taijiquan helps the hip pain.

我在 2005 年向何医生学太极拳，我喜欢每天清晨在院前，（在一个树木繁茂的农村地区）练拳，我感到很高兴地活着。我有髋关节问题，也约了星期四看针灸师，星期三晚上练太极拳，星期四髋关节就没痛了。

我认为太极拳有助于缓解髋关节疼痛。

75. Less Pain and Stiffness
减轻疼痛和僵硬

By Rosemary Britt

Taijiquan helped me feel stronger and more flexible in my body. After doing *Taijiquan* for six weeks I feel less pain and stiffness in my neck and back. *Taijiquan* has helped me with my focus and concentration and even improved my memory to study for school. I feel more relaxed and also energized. Thank you for sharing *Taijiquan* with me. I enjoy doing *Taijiquan* better in a class setting than by myself.

In the future, I would like to continue classes.

在练习太极拳的 6 个星期里，我感到脖子和背部的疼痛和僵硬减轻了。太极拳帮助了我的注意力集中，甚至提高了我的记忆力，方便学习。我感到更加轻松，也充满了活力。谢谢分享太极拳。我喜欢在课堂上一起练太极拳，感到比自己一人做更好。

在未来，我要继续上太极拳课。

76. The Importance Of Taijiquan
太极拳的重要性

By Tricia L. Mattson

As a student at the American Academy of Acupuncture and Oriental Medicine, I have to take *Taijiquan* for the program. Before starting about a month ago, I had had friends try to teach me *Taijiquan*,and always wanted to learn more about it.

Being the very busy person that I am, I find that my biggest challenge with the exercises is slowing down and focusing. There are times that I get so frustrated with myself that I want to leave the class. However, it is in these moments that I realize the importance of *Taijiquan* and why I feel so good after class.

Moreover, by forcing myself to focus and slow down I become a better student and person.

我是一个美国针灸和东方医学（美国中医学院）的学生，太极拳是必修课。在开始学的一个月前，我曾经请我的朋友尝试教我太极拳，想要更加的了解它。

作为非常忙碌的人，我觉得练习太极拳最大的挑战是放慢速度和集中注意力。好几次，我对自己感到泄气，我不想上这门课了。然而，正是这时刻让我意识到太极拳的重要性。

上完太极拳课后我感觉如此良好。此外，强迫自己集中注意力和放慢速度，可以让我成为一个更好的学生和更好的人。

77. Taijiquan And My Fate
太极拳与我的命运

By Meredith Wodrich

I have only been studying *Taijiquan* for 9 weeks. However, I had a strange experience with *Taijiquan* that started 20 years ago. Back then, I had a dream one night that I walked into a travel agency office. I was looking at brochures of travel in Tibet and China. Suddenly, there was a man standing in front of me (a Tibetan monk, I think). He reached out a hand to me and the gesture sent me flying backward across the room! When I woke up, I knew I was somehow being called (to China), but I was not sure what.

Now, 20 years later, I am a student of TCM（Traditional Chinese medicine）at AAAOM. In one class, we watched a file of a story on *Taijiquan* masters. One master does with his students exactly what I experienced in my dream! Then, I knew I was in the right place.

Since starting *Taijiquan*, I have already noticed changes. I feel calm and alert and clearly see improvement in my balance! My body takes to it naturally. I feel my mind is empty and floating while I do *Taijiquan*. I love it!!

我只学了太极拳9周。我对太极拳有一种奇怪的经历，是20年前在台湾开始的。那时，一天晚上我做了一个梦，我走进一家旅行社的办公室。我看着去西藏和中国旅游的小册子。突然，有一个人站在我的面前（我想是一位藏族僧人）。他伸出手给我，那手势让我向后飞到房间的另一端。当我醒来的时候，不知怎么被召唤到了一个叫中国的地方，我不确定是怎么回事。

现在，20年后，我是在美国中医学院学（AAAOM）习中医的学生。上课时，我们看了一个有关太极拳师父的故事，这就是我所经历的梦境。然后，我知道自己来到了正确的地方。

自练太极拳之后，我已注意到一些变化。我感到平静和清醒，并清楚地看到我的平衡能力的改善。我的身体自然的接受它。在练太极拳时我觉得我的头脑是空灵的。我爱太极拳！

78. Pull May Seat Belt 拉安全带

By Elizabeth Clark

A short story from someone who is new to *Taijiquan* and has just learned the 24 Form. I recently bought a different car, and had been trying to figure out how to reach where the top of the seat belt was connected so that I could pull it forward without over-stretching—it always seemed just beyond my reach.

Then one day last week as I turned to reach back, my eyes followed my hand as I turned it palm up, just like in the "Step Back and Repulse the Monkey" form.

Voila! I easily reached the seat belt.

这是一个刚学过 24 式太极拳的小故事。我最近才买了一部车子，我一直在试图弄清楚如何够到安全带顶部的连接位置，这样我要将它向前拉而不需要过度拉伸—它似乎总是在我够不到的地方。才拉得起来。

上个礼拜某一天，我转过身来拉安全带，眼随手走手心朝上，犹如太极拳"倒卷猴"动作。

瞧！太极拳帮我轻松地拉到了安全带。

79. Learn To Ride Bicycle 学会骑自行车

By Li Hongxia

I tried to learn to ride a bicycle many times but have not succeeded, because whenever I try to ride the bicycle leans and falls.

Since I learned *Taijiquan* it was much better. When I am practicing and lose my balance while riding the bicycle again, I just practice *Taijiquan*. Then my balance is fine; the bicycle does not lean sideways, and I am able to ride it!

I am glad I finally learned to ride a bicycle with the help of *Taijiquan*.

我学了好多次自行车也没有学会，因为一骑车，车就歪倒了。自学了太极拳就好多了，我在练车时，车不平衡又要倒了，於是我马上练太极拳，平衡就好了，车不侧倾了，我也就能骑上去了。

我很高兴终于在太极拳的帮助下学会了骑自行车。

80. More at Peace 更加平静

By Mallory Carlson

I have been practicing *Taijiquan* for about 2 months and I have noticed a marked difference in my general mood and attitude. I feel more at peace and I have more patience with others and potentially frustrating situations.

Physically, I am also more relaxed. It is encouraging; while I am doing *Taijiquan* it has subtle manifestations, for example, my palms become distinctly warmer.

我已经练了太极拳二个月了，我注意到我的心情和态度有了显著的变化。我觉得更加平静，我对别人和可能令人沮丧的情况时有更多的耐心。

我的身体也更放松了。令人鼓舞的是当我打太极拳的时候，它微妙的现象显现出来，如我手掌明确的变暖就是一个例子。

81. Focus, and Relax 专注和放松

By Julie Muduy

I really like how centered, focused, and relaxed I feel after doing *Taijiquan*. My brain feels good and balanced.

我真的很喜欢练习完太极拳后那种专注、思想集中和放松的感觉。我的感觉很好，身体平衡。

82. Help Me with Energy 帮助我有能量

By Marco Yecuiai

I started doing *Taijiquan* 6 years ago. I was surprised, no matter how bad my condition was before doing *Taijiquan*, I felt good afterward, especially when I am tired, it helps me with energy. It also helps my joints become more flexible.

6 年前我开始练太极拳。我很惊讶，不管我练太极拳之前多么糟糕，练完太极拳后确实感到变好，尤其在累时，太极拳帮助我有能量，也让我的关节更有柔韧性。

83. Feel Good Life 感到生活美好

By Ye Yang

Before I played Taijiquan, I had trouble getting good sleep at night. I dreamed too much and felt restless and tired the next morning. I looked pale on the face and felt tired inside.

However, after I started to play Taijiquan every day for 20 minutes, my sleep improved a lot. Ten weeks after, my hands and feet started to warm, and my face got its first hue. The best thing is that it improves my mood and energy, and makes me feel good about life and work.

在我练太极拳前，睡眠不好，而且多梦，第二天起床很累。我的脸色苍白，身体总是感到疲倦。

但每天练太极拳 20 分钟后睡眠好，十个礼拜后，我手足温暖起来，脸色有光泽。最好的是太极拳帮助我了的心情和精力，让我对生活和工作感觉良好。

84. Taijiquan Makes My Blood Sugar and Pressure Levels are Back to Normal 太极拳使我的血糖和血压正常

By Wu Jiayi

During the war, the difficult living conditions caused me to develop a gastric ulcer. Ever since, I always suffered from stomachaches, low appetite, and sometimes had blood in my stool. In 1985, I was diagnosed with coronary artery disease, low blood pressure, spurs in my cervical vertebrae, and bronchitis. At that time, I was almost 60 years old and I thought that there would be no hope for me for the rest of my life. My mood went down to the bottom, and I was depressed all the time. For about 3 years I had to walk with a cane, and I even passed out several times at work. I visited many big hospitals, but the treatment results were not good.

Starting in 1986, I started to learn Yang-style *Taijiquan* and *Taijisword* for an hour every day. A year later, the GI exam I had showed that the gastric ulcer was partially recovered. Now I am less stressed and have not had coronary artery disease for three years. My neck no longer hurts. My blood sugar and blood pressure levels are back to normal. I do not cough anymore and haven't been in a hospital in 4 years.

Before, my feet and legs were very weak, and I had a hard time with balance when walking. Sometimes when I was in a crowded market, I dared not move! After I started exercising *Taijiquan*, my energy level went up, and I can go wherever I want without being frightened!

I am energetic all the time and no longer have depression or anxiety. I can work not only harder but also smarter with increased efficiency. Although I am in my sixties right now, I feel much younger and life is full of hope. My friends even call me "old youth" sometimes.

I believe all these changes happened because *Taijiquan* is exhibiting its magic power on me!

在战争年代，因为生活艰苦紧张，患了十二指肠球部溃疡。长期胃疼，食欲不振，不时便血，身体虚弱。1985 年又患了神经衰弱，冠心病，低血压，颈椎骨质增生，支气管炎等病。当时，我刚近 60 岁，就半死不活的，心情极其忧郁。有 3 年多时间，我都是扶着拐杖走路，曾几次昏倒，我曾多次到重庆和成都求医，但疗效不佳。

1986 年我开始学杨式太极拳，太极剑，每天 1 小时。一年后经胃镜检查，"十二指肠球部溃疡部分愈合"，神经衰弱也好了，冠心病已 3 年内多未复发。颈部不痛，血糖，血压基本正常，也不再咳嗽了，已四年多未住院了。过去我因双脚无力，走路不稳，一遇赶集人多，我就不敢动弹。练拳几年后，力气大增，赶集天人再多再挤，我也无所畏惧了。

现在，我心情开朗精力充沛，脑子清醒苦脑全无，不但能整日坚持工作，而且工作效率大大提高，虽然我已年满 6 旬，却感到青春焕发，越活越有劲。朋友们都叫我"老青年"。

我相信这一切的变化都是因为太极拳在我身上展示了它的魔力！

85. Help Me Calm 帮助平静

By Caroline Collins

I had no previous experience with Taijiquan before taking Dr. He's class. I always felt more calm and more relaxed after class no matter how stressed I was when I walked in. Near the end of this trimester, when we were more comfortable with the sequence and would go through it as a group, the energy in the room felt like it really grew and expanded. It was one of my favorite things about this class.

All of the teachers were wonderful, very knowledgeable, entertaining, and patient. Thank you!

我在上何大夫的课之前没有太极拳的经历。不管我走进练太极拳的教室时压力有多大，下太极拳课后我会觉得平静和放松。这学期接近尾声，当我们已更熟练这些动作，并和大家一起练习时，真的感到能量在增长和扩大。这是我上课最喜欢的事情之一。

所有的老师都非常的好，富有知识，有趣和有耐心。谢谢！

86. Made Me Dance More Graceful
让我跳舞更优美

By Mary Rian

I have been practicing *Taijiquan* since class started in January 2005. I felt its effects immediately! *Taijiquan* has helped me to relax and stay focused in this very challenging first trimester back in school. It has also helped me in my dance classes (West African). I find that I am more graceful and coordinated, I have been dancing for 10 years and I noticed a difference! *Taijiquan* has helped me balance my life in many ways.

I am very happy that I have found it!

我从 2005 年 1 月开始开始练习太极拳。我立刻就感受到了它的效果！太极拳帮助我放松，让我在这个非常具有挑战性的三个月保持专注。它帮助了我的舞蹈课（西非舞）。我已经跳舞 10 年了，我发现我跳舞更优雅，更协调，更有长进了。我还注意到了一个不同，太极拳帮助了我很多方面，平衡了我的生活。

我很高兴我找到了它！

87. More Focused 更加专注

By Pam Bailey

I have done aerobic exercise my entire life and have been doing yoga and sitting meditation consistently for over 5 years. In sitting meditation, the mind has a tendency to wander off, because there is nothing concrete for it to focus on. In yoga, you move into a posture and hold it; again, the mind has a chance to wander off. But in *Taijiquan*, the mind must focus on the constant movement and changing positions of the body. If the mind wanders off, you'll lose your place in the sequence of movements.

When I practice *Taijiquan*, I am very mindful and aware with less effort.

I also think that *Taijiquan* improves physical strength, balance, and agility. I am active but not very athletic or graceful. When practicing *Taijiquan*, I feel my body moving slowly and smoothly, as if I'm dancing. My body feels rhythmic and flowing; my mind feels calm and centered.

我做了一辈子的有氧运动，并一直练瑜伽和打坐冥想5年多了。在打坐冥想时，注意力会有种偏离的倾向，因为没有什么具体东西可以关注。做瑜伽时，做了一个动作就保持不动，再做一次，注意力便乘机溜走了。但练习太极拳，必须关注身体的持续运动和变化的位置。如果头脑偏离了，你就会忘掉动作。因此当我练习太极拳时，我不必费吹灰之力就能非常专注，练太极拳比练瑜伽更能专注。

我还认为，太极拳提高体力，平衡和灵活性。我很活跃，但不是很擅长运动，也不优雅。当练太极拳时，我感觉我的身体运动缓慢而平稳，就好像我在跳舞。我的身体感觉有韵律和流畅；我的头脑感到平静和集中。

88. Improve the Immune System
提高免疫系统

By Peter Laudert

I began learning Taijiquan 19 years ago after witnessing an impressive demonstration of Taijiquan martial applications. My interest in Taijiquan was mainly for its use as a martial art - I was not really aware of its health benefits. But as the years passed I began to realize that, gosh, I haven't been sick for a really long time.

Taijiquan boosts the immune system, and I haven't had a serious illness since learning Taijiquan, or even a cold or the flu for many years. Taijiquan has also been very beneficial for relieving stress and increasing my emotional harmony. It's really been a blessing.

19年前，我目睹了一个令人印象深刻的太极拳武术应用的演示后，开始学习太极拳。我对太极拳的兴趣主要是由于它作为一种武术——我并不真正知道它对健康的好处。但随着时间的流逝，我开始意识到，天哪，我已经很久没有生病了。

太极拳可以增强免疫系统，自从学习太极拳后，我多年来就没有患过严重的疾病，甚至是感冒或流感。太极拳也对缓解压力和增加情绪平和很有好处，这真是一种幸事。

89. True Meditation 真正的冥想

By Myra Fishman

I had forgotten the movements since I had last taken Dr. He's class eight years ago and therefore decided to re-enroll.

I find that the deep concentration that *Taijiquan* requires, offers me the opportunity to attain self-wellness. I have found that my balance has improved dramatically, along with my strength as well. The warm-up exercises and the *Taijiquan* movements have been extremely helpful in improving bone density and relieving pain and discomfort in my neck, back, and hips.

Taijiquan movements coupled with timed breaths are true meditation for me. As an extra bonus, I feel truly relaxed and refreshed afterward. *Taijiquan* is very important to me. I fully intend to continue to incorporate *Taijiquan* into my daily routine.

我忘记了 8 年前上何大夫的太极拳课，因此我决定重新注册。

我觉得太极拳要求的深度精神集中，让我有机会帮助自己的健康。平衡和力量都有大的改善。热身练习和太极拳运动一直非常的有助于改善骨质密度，减轻疼痛，缓解脖子、背部和臀部的不适感。

太极拳动作配合呼吸对我来说是真正的冥想，还让我真正的放松和焕然一新。我完全打算继续把太极拳融入到我的日常生活中。

90.Help Balance And Deep Breathing
帮助平衡和深呼吸

By Brandy Trinz

Just practicing Taijiquan in class over the course of two class segments has really improved two aspects of my well-being. The first is balance. When I began classes, I could not do the postures on one leg or do the kicking moves very easily. After practicing, I can now do the move on one leg without losing balance, and the kicking motion is much easier.

The second aspect that has improved is my ability to do deep breathing. The techniques Dr. He has shown us for breathing in and filling our bellies with air and then emptying our bellies breathing out (much the opposite of how we often are taught to breath) have increased my capacity for deep breathing for meditation or just to relax when I'm tensing up. Thanks much!

只在课堂上练了太极拳近 2 个课程，就让我身体的两种状况更好了。第一是平衡，当我开始学习时我并不能轻易地做好独脚站立或蹬腿。在练习之后我可以很容易地做好独脚站立，和蹬腿。

第二件事是增强了我做深呼吸的能力，何大夫教了我们吸气时让空气充满我们的肚子，然后吐气时把肚子的气吐空（这和我们平时被教的方法非常不同）有助于我去深度的呼气去帮助我冥想或紧张时助我放松。

91. Reliance on Taijiquan Brings Peace & Eases Headaches
太极拳带来平静和缓解头痛

By Terry Connors

I've been participating Taijiquan as taught by Dr. He,for less than one year, yet I've already come to rely upon the tranquility that each session brings to me. Taijiquan has been tremendously helpful as I contend with many mid-life transitions. It also eases headaches!

我参加何医生的太极拳班虽然不到一年，但我已经开始依赖每一次练习给我带来的平静。太极拳对我非常有用，因为我要应对许多中年期的过渡。此外太极拳还能缓解头痛！

92. Enjoy the Peace 享受平静

By Carol

I really enjoy the peace and serenity I feel when I do Taijiquan. It helps me to focus on my breathing and helps me to clear my head. The slowness of the movement helps me to remember to slow down in my every day life and in my recovery.

I often find myself rushing through my day and Taijiquan helps me focus and be more mindful and stay in the present. It has been an amazing exercise to help me clear my mind and worry with less which greatly helps in my recovery.

我真的很享受打太极拳时的平静和宁静。它帮助我专注于我的呼吸，帮助我清醒。动作的缓慢帮助我在我的日常生活中慢下来。

我经常发现自己每天都在匆忙中度过，太极拳能帮助我集中注意力，更专注，活在当下。这是一个神奇的锻炼，帮助我清理我的头脑和担心更少，大大有助于我身体的恢复。

93. I Want to Practice Taijiquan Consistently 坚持练习太极拳

By Zheng Zhen

Taijiquan in traditional Chinese culture is a unique sport; it includes martial arts, Qigong, and fitness in one, and is becoming more and more loved by many people all over the world.

Dr. He inherited her late father's last wish: to make every effort to spread Chinese *Taijiquan* culture in the United States. Her will is commendable, her affection moves me, and her action is admirable. As one of her students, I am much honored to be taught by Dr. He. Her father is a great Taijiquan master. Under the careful guidance of Dr. He, I learned systematically, and steadily enjoyed and learned the essence of *Taijiquan*. It has valuable insights, a physical and psychological boost, and the body becomes increasingly strong.

I am grateful for Dr. He's lectures, and I am determined to keep practicing *Taijiquan*, to achieve "fist never leaves the hand" [a proverb meaning skill only comes with constant practice]. Through this I will make my life one of high quality and continue to live that way. I think every person desires this.

太极拳是中国传统文化所独有的一种运动，她集武术、气功和健身于一体，越来越得到世界广大人民的喜爱。

何医生继承其先父的意志，努力将中华太极拳文化在美国传播，其志可嘉，其情感人，其行令人敬佩。我做为学生中的一员，能得到何老师的教导（她的父亲就是一个很棒的太极拳大师），真是荣幸之至。在何医生的精心指导下，我从一招一式学起，逐步品尝和吸取太极拳的精义，真是感悟良多，身心振奋，身体也日趋强壮。

感激何医生的教导，我决心坚持练习太极拳，做到《拳不离手》，使自己的生命以高质量的方式显现和延续。我想这也是每一个人所期望的。

94. The Benefits of Practicing Taijiquan
练习太极拳的好处

By HJ Chen

In 1999, I went to University of Minnsota with my two children to learn Taijiquan from Uncle He. After that, we invited Uncle He to our house as a gust for few weeks. Every morning, Uncle He led us to practice Taijiquan in our backyard, and two kids also followed . We were practicing the classic Taijiquan with 118 forms.

Practicing Taijiquan can relax the body! Relax mind! Every morning I practice Taijiquan after warm up body by swim my arms and rotating my waist. Taijiquan 118 forms are long. The older age I get, the harder to remember the order of all the movements. But, I still can practice it smoothly. Turn waist left and right. Foot step leads by the direction of the waist. Rotate the waist and spine, and using the power of the waist to drive the arms. If the next movement was forgotten, I just continue with any form which can be followed smoothly, and move on. Finally, at the end, do the closing form and complete the practice. At that time, Uncle Ho also taught us how to use those movements in real fighting. During my own practicing, I'm trying to imitate each offense and defense movements learn from Uncle Ho. This help me to practice Taijiquan more smoothly.

After practice Taijiquan, the body feel relaxed! And the reaction becomes quicker. However, I realize that in addition to practice the movements and rotate the waist, we should also improve strength of the legs! For example, one can practice Squat horse step! Once the strength of the legs are well developed, we'll not easy to fall!

There are many benefits to practicing Taijiquan in older age! But want to get the real benefit, one must pursue unremittingly.

1999 年我带著两个孩子到明大随著何伯伯学习太极拳。后来，我們特地邀請何伯伯到家里做客数週。何伯伯每天早上在后院帶我們一起练习太极拳，两个孩子也都一起跟着。当时练的是 118 式。

练习太极拳可以让身体放松，心情放松！所以，我每天清早都会先甩甩手、转转腰熱身后，打一趟太极拳。

118 式很長，年紀愈長，愈来愈不易記住全部招式的順序，但是，仍然可以打得流暢！左右轉腰、步隨腰轉！轉腰旋脊，用腰来帶手臂！后面招式忘了，就用可以順勢的一招接续下去。最后，合太极、收式。当时，何伯伯也教我們如何运用那些招式。我也在练习太极拳时去体会每一式如何拆招应敌！这也让我在练习时，打得更易流暢。

年纪大了，练习太极拳确有很多好处！但是要持之以恆，必有益处！

95. Saves Money and Ensure Own Life
省钱和保命

Forget-me-not

I have been learning Taijiquan from Doctor He for several months, It feels like it helps a lot.

1. Save money and save time.

I used to reduce stress by driving fast on the highway for 40 minutes every night. Now just practice Taijiquan, Relax for just 10 minutes. Save money on gas, Reduced car wear and tear.

2. To ensure own life safety.

Driving fast on the highway.Life is hard to protect.There was a car accident, Broken arm or leg is no fun.I can keep my life at home, and make oneself relaxed and happy.

3. Reduce environmental pollution.

I'm smart enough, Is that right？

Friends envied me, then practice Taijiquan quickly！

我跟随何医生学习太极拳已经好几个月了，感觉很有用。

1. 省钱省时。过去我减轻压力是每天晚上在高速公路上飙车40分钟。现在练习太极拳，仅仅10分钟就可以放松自己。节省了汽油费，减少了汽车的磨损，还节约了时间。

2. 保障了自己的生命安全。在高速公路上狂飙，小命很难保。出了车祸，断了胳膊、腿不好玩。在家就可以保命，还让自己轻松愉快。

3. 减少环境污染。

我很聪明，对吗？

朋友们羡慕我吗？那么就赶快练太极拳吧！

96.Taijiquan to Be Calming
太极拳能让人平静

By Kathy

It is more than 20 years ago when I went to Dr. He the first time for acupuncture because of a problematic health condition. After treating me, she happened to mention that she would soon be starting a new session of Taijiquan classes, and recommended I take them, because stress was contributing to my problem.

Since then, I've retaken the class with Dr He once or twice, took Dr. He's Qi Gong classes, and have gone to many of the monthly practice sessions, which I find very helpful. Taijiquan makes me much more aware of the energy in my body, and balances that energy.

I find Taijiquan to be calming and at the same time gently energizing. The monthly practice group is made up of friendly people, and I enjoy going to reconnect with them. I had a local neighborhood group I could practice with more regularly. Group practice helps me remember the sequence.

I am very grateful for Dr. He and all that I have learned from her, which includes learning a few words of Chinese! Dr. He is smart, kind, funny and is a wise and revered teacher.

那是 20 多年前，因为健康问题，我去看何医生，第一次做针灸。在治疗我之后，碰巧提到她很快就会开始一个新的太极课程，并建议我上，因为压力导致了我的问题。

从那以后，我又重新跟何医生上了一两次太极课程，还上了何医生的气功课。并参加了许多次每个月的复习课，这很有帮助。太极拳让我更意识到身体的能量，平衡。

我发现太极给人平静，同时也很温和，充满活力。每月的练习小组是由友好的人组成的，我很喜欢与他们重新联系。我有一个当地的社区团体，我可以经常地和他们一起练习。小组练习帮助我记住了太极拳的顺序。

我非常感谢何医生和从她那里学到的一切，其中包括学习几个汉语单词！何医生聪明、善良、风趣，是一位充满智慧而受人尊敬的老师。

97. Taijiquan Experience 太极拳的体验

By James Postiglione, 7th-Generation Lineage holder

A difficult task before me 一个艰巨的任务摆在我面前
To describe my Taijiquan experience 描述我的太极拳经历
Something so important, 这么重要的东西，
Such a part of me 就像我身体的一部分
Something started by chance, 一次偶然的开始，
Perhaps a hobby, no thought of more 或许是嗜好，没多想
Two teachers provide a taste 两位老师提供了一个体验
Then with Sifus Ray and Paul so much more 然后雷和保罗师父给
我更深的体验
Through poor health and good 从体弱多病到良好的健康
Practice, repetition and guidance 反复的练习和咨询
A feeling grows, 一种感觉在增长，
Subtlety changing flesh and spirit 是肉体和精神的微妙变化
Blood flow felt, 感到血液的流动，
breath lowered, 呼吸降低，
legs strengthened, 腿部坚挺，
sinews unraveled 筋骨放松
Agitation ever present 烦乱一直都在
aggressive reaction decreases 暴躁的反应降低
learn to wait, be still 学会等待，静下心来
a solution is found 定会找到解决方案
Universal energy felt, 感到宇宙能量，

connection to heaven and earth once again 再次连接天地

Collisions sensed, averted 遇到冲突、选择避开

Intensity diffused 强烈的感情消散

Danger present, 在当前的危险中,

Safety found 找到平安

Progress is rapid, then slow 进步是快的，然后是慢的

First small gains are measured in days 几天的练习之后，第一批小收获

Months turn to years before whole body connected 长年累月的练习之后，身心灵合一

Many levels hoped for some day 希望有一天能达到更高水平

Time is precious, demands endless 时间宝贵，学无止境

Choices are many 选择有很多

Taijiquan brings great rewards 太极拳带来丰厚的回报

What value can there be on health? 它对健康有什么价值？

On 20 minutes of peace?20 分钟的心平气和？

On feeling inner chi? 感觉内在的气？

On being centered and connected? 感觉平衡和心灵合一？

With practice rewards are many-fold 随着训练，必以倍数回报。

98. Less Chance of Falling 减少摔跤

Kam Keung Kam

My name is Kam Keung Kam. I have the privilege to learn Tai Chi Chuan from Master Ming He and Dr. XinRong He in Twin City, Minnesota. Since then, I have practiced some of the movements regularly. I am beneficial from practicing Tai Chi Chuan in becoming more peaceful, healthier, and less chance of falling

我的名字是甘鑑强。我有幸从明尼苏达州双城的何明大师及何新蓉博士那里学习太极拳。从那时起，我就定期练习一些动作。练习太极拳有利于我变得更平静，更健康，还减少了跌倒的机会。

L. Commemorative Articles for Mr. He Ming by Relatives & Friends 亲友们纪念何明老先生

99. Recollections of Taijiquan 太极拳往事

Gong Changzhen, Ph.D. 博士

After a person has lived over half of his or her life learning knowledge and skills and receiving advice from renowned experts and mentors, it might look like showing off if he or she mentions those big names to others. Actually, I think that is not always the case. I think mentioning or in acknowledging is to show respect to those famous experts and teachers. In fact, I feel even more strongly about this as time elapses. Every time I said the names of my professors or mentors, it always felt like encouragement—as if they were there with me. While I was studying and teaching mathematics for ten years at Shandong University in China, I attended classes instructed by academicians and famous mathematicians. They were either residential at Shandong University or visiting professors from other institutes. Later I devoted my time towards economics, where I spent five years pursuing my Ph.D. at the University of Minnesota. I studied with the superstars in economics who later become Nobel Prize winners in economics. Then, my interest had transitioned to acupuncture and Chinese medicine where I met and learned from numerous national grand masters and famous experts. In this recollection article, I am not talking about those mathematics academicians, nor the Nobel Prize winners in economics, but rather I am speaking about a person who influenced me greatly on Taijiquan, and more generally on my mind-body exercises. This person is Mr. He Ming. Getting to know Mr. He Ming not only transformed my perception of

Taijiquan into a healthy exercise, but also led me to explore medical Qi Gong, such as Yi Jin Jing, Liu Zi Jue and Wu Qin Xi. From there, I started to not only value these exercises but it led me to embark on a life-long journey.

The first time I met Mr. He Ming was in 1995. When Dr. He Xinrong, Mr. He Ming's daughter, decided to stay in the United States to join my effort to develop Chinese medicine in the United States, Mr. He Ming visited Minnesota. The first encounter with Mr. He Ming left a huge impression. He had a thin face filled with kindness and wisdom. His face carried all his life's vicissitudes. He was eighty-five years old. He had an upright back and walked swiftly. His eyes were bright. He responded very quickly. I respected him immensely as he was a graduate of Whampoa Military Academy. As a witness to the stormy history of both the Republic of China and the People's Republic of China, Mr. He was full of extraordinary wisdom and rich thoughts. Taijiquan Quan accompanied Mr. He Ming for his life. He had taught over 20000 Tai Ji students for over 67 years in Chongqing, all of whom had benefited greatly. So naturally, when Mr. He Ming came to the United States he also brought with him Tai Ji Quan.

It was a scene I'll never forget. The first clinic of our TCM Health Center was established in 1995 in the University Technology Center office building adjacent to the University of Minnesota. The activity center hall of this office building was located in the middle of the first floor of the building. The hall was two floors high, so the lights were very high on the ceiling. From the east and west sides of the hall, you could see the sky and the stars outside through the huge window glass. This hall could hold 200 people for meetings, but only 50 people could practice Taijiquan.

One side (the north side) of the hall had a podium raised above the ground. The rostrum was set up from east to west, crossing the

244

entire hall. Every Wednesday night, the music was playing, Mr. He Ming wore a loose plain Taijiquan suit made of white hemp, and Dr. He Xinrong wore a light pink silk Taijiquan suit. Mr. He Ming and Dr. He Xinrong elegantly demonstrated the " White Crane Spreads its Wings", "Wild Horse Separates Mane", "Golden Rooster Stands on its One Leg" on the rostrum, and more than 40 students followed Mr. He and Dr. He's beautiful movements. Students were very concentrated. The local newspaper, Asia American Press, sent reporter Ms. S. A. Lucas to interview Mr. He during Taijiquan numerous times.

Mr. He Ming could only speak a few English words and couldn't communicate with American students fluently, but this did not seem to be a barrier between them at all. After each Taijiquan class, a few students always surrounded him and asked questions, as if they spoke the same language. In addition, he had a unique skill. As long as he felt that the students' questions were about Taijiquan, he would answer them with Taijiquan demonstrations. Mr. He turned the movements and postures of Taijiquan into the universal language of the world. What a lovely old gentleman!

Mr. He Ming stayed in my home several times. Every time he was staying at housewhen the sun rose, Mr. He Ming added a landscape to my backyard. My backyard is shaded by a dense forest. Decades-old maple trees, oaks, iron trees, and poplar trees stretch up into the clouds and surround my backyard. Every morning, as the sun slanted through the woods from the east into my backyard, Mr. He Ming had already started to practice his Taijiquan On the green lawn, the vigorous old man was already doing " Hands Play P'i P'a", " Brush Knee and Push Step", and " Strike the Ears with Double Fists ". The chirping of birds on the surrounding trees was accompanied by the music of Mr. He Ming's Taijiquan. Those graceful postures of stillness in movement and movement in stillness were completely blended into nature.

After finishing Taijiquan every morning, Mr. He Ming sat down to take his notes. His notebook was full of what was happening and his comments. He recorded all the interesting things we discussed. There were also reports from Chinese newspapers "World Daily" and "Xing Dao Daily", which he cut out and pasted onto his notebook.

In the days when Mr. He Ming lived in my house, he also transcribed "Cai Gen Tan" every day. It happened to be when he was transcribing "Cai Gen Tan" and reciting those famous lines, I had a deeper understanding about "when nothing happened, keep the mind clear, when something happened, be very cautious," "For a person without excessive desire for material things, it is like the autumn sky without clouds and huge ocean with quietness; For a person pursuing a peaceful life, as long as dulcimer and books are available, it is like living in a paradise", " When you are free, don't let go of your precious time, it will be useful when you are busy; when you are calm, don't forget to enrich your spirit, and you will be able to cope with the heavy responsibilities; don't do bad things even when no one knows; if you do everything above board, you will be respected in the public", "what happened in the outside world should not be taken very seriously". An old man who had won so much respect was the true embodiment of these lines.

Self-massage and meditation were added into our Taijiquan class. Students sat quietly to calm their spirit, focused on the Dantian. Self-massaging Zusanli, Sanyinjiao, and Neiguan were practiced during the break between the two half sessions. The class ended with Shiatsu Anmian point, pressing Taichong and Hegu. Countless patients and students have benefited immensely from these mind-body exercises with Eastern wisdom.

I once took Mr. He Ming and my family to the University of

Minnesota Arboretum, and he showed great interest in the flowers, trees, streams, and ponds there. Lindens, maples, ash trees, and locust trees are arranged with order and intention. On the grass next to the hawthorn trees and crabapple trees, Mr. He Ming led us to practice Taijiquan. Not only did our actions attract some park visitors, but the squirrels all around stood up and looked at us. After Mr. He Ming finished a short form of Taijiquan, he said, "Look, the squirrel also wanted to practice Taijiquan!"

Mr. He Ming had visited Minnesota several times and had always left with a deep and good impression on Minnesota. In 1999, I organized a special trip to visit New York. Because of our large group including my father, Dr. Gu Li and his wife Mrs. Shang Jin, we stayed in a family hotel run by a woman from Shanghai. The landlord acclaimed New York as much as she praised her hometown Shanghai. The landlord in her 60s exclaimed with great pride that New York is a very exciting city, from the famous Statue of Liberty to all kinds of festivities to even the busy traffic and to the non-stop neon lights at night. She believed all the stimulants made it so that nobody suffered from Alzheimer's disease there. She compared New York to a piece of stinky tofu that smells and tastes delicious. Mr. He Ming immediately replied Minnesota has the largest lake in North America. Minnesota was like a steamed bread with white flour. It tastes delicious and smells more fragrant. The more you chew, the more delicious it is. Everyone laughed. The swiftness of Mr. He Ming's response was astonishing, his responsiveness was highly commendable, and his humorous responses expressed his deep affection for Minnesota.

In 1999, the American Academy of Traditional Chinese Medicine officially opened. Dr. He Xinrong was the teacher of the Taijiquan class. Mr. He Ming came again from Chongqing to co-teach the class. In fact, many students in the Taijiquan class were not students of our traditional Chinese medicine school who intended to earn a degree, but rather the patients of our clinic or family members and friends who had been introduced by the patients. Taijiquan classes and Qi Gong classes were the only classes open to the public and the community among all the courses in the school of traditional Chinese medicine. Many Taijiquan class students also came to learn from Mr. He Ming because of his reputation. There were some students who drove seven to eight hours from Chicago and the Canadian borders to join our class. From 1995 to 1999, Mr. He Ming came to the United States for Taijiquan classes many times, and many students wanted to be followers and some even became Mr. He Ming's biggest fans. When they heard that Mr. He continued to teach the class, and with each passing year many old students came to review. The Taijiquan class was always growing and our class continued to be held in the event center of the building.

Mr. He Ming gave great enthusiasm to our newly opened acupuncture and Chinese medicine college. At that time, Dr. Gu Li had just left Los Angeles to come to Minnesota to join our group. Mr. He Ming not only continued to teach our Taijiquan class with Dr. He Xinrong, but also helped us fold brochures and put stamps on them for recruiting new students. The enthusiasm of Mr. He Ming was evidenced by a poem he left:

Ode to Taoyuan
March 10, 1999
Taoyuan is a legend for ages,
It is happening to the present.
Liu and Gong's friendship and love,
Comparable to emperor's uncle Liu.
Gu and He's passion and loyalty,
Superior to Zhang and Guan.

All wishes come true,

Following the bright light.

Three families work for one goal,

Making effort with one heart.

Six gentlemen raised their arms,

to beat the drum.

Without achieving the goal,

The drum will not stop.

Unexpectedly, when Mr. He Ming left these passionate lines, it was only about six months before the end of his life. On October 28, 1999, Mr. He Ming left us forever. He left us so peacefully, so calmly, without burdening his children and without any suffering himself. His optimism and being fondness for learning new things left a legacy for us. We continued the Taijiquan class that Mr. He Ming left us to this day and I wish we could forever. Every once in a while, I always think of that kind of old man. On the tenth anniversary of Mr. He Ming's death, I wrote a poem to commemorate:

A Tribute to Mr.He Ming

October 2009

Thousands of trees are scattered,

Lakes are covered by smokes and clouds.

Lonely goose is circling,

It is ready to start a southern tour.

All buildings are still there,

Stands on the setting sun.

It rains in the autumn every year,

The late person is remembered.

Time is fleeting,
Ten springs and autumns come and go.
The integrity and fortitude remain.
Taijiquan's lesson not forgotten,
Gratefulness to the dead,
Is in my heart.

Twenty years had passed by October 2019 and our school of traditional Chinese medicine not only established a Master of Acupuncture program and a Master of Traditional Chinese Medicine program but also established a Doctor of Traditional Chinese Medicine program. At this critical moment, I thought of Mr. He Ming who taught me personally and gave me great emotional support and encouragement. I once again wrote a poem to express my recollections:

A Reminiscence to Mr. He Ming
October 2019
Clear water,
Blue sky,
Red maple leaves,
Goose moans,
Echoed across the sky.
In the middle of the night,
The moon tilts westward,
Longing for past is speechless
I fear to bolt the heaven.

Heroic spirits remain

In the Jialing River,

Dreams are surrounding

The Mississippi River.

Taijiquan students should not be ungrateful,

The past memory is like a smoke

But stays for life.

These little poems were just my own memorial to Mr. He Ming. When it comes to remembrance, it's not just mine. More than 20 years ago, when Mr. He Ming brought Taijiquan to Minnesota, nobody took Taijiquan as a medical treatment. Just after Taijiquan was widely spread, American medical schools and medical centers began to push Taijiquan into the medical arena. This may be the greatest consolation for Mr. He Ming's spirit in heaven. The poems left by Mr. He and my memorial have been kept with two medical journals. The two medical journals are the 2010 and 2012 issues of the New England Journal of Medicine. In these two medical journals, two clinical randomized controlled trials of Taijiquan conducted by American scientists were published. The two studies were trials for treating patients with fibromyalgia syndrome and Parkinson's disease, respectively.

Fibromyalgia has become a common condition affecting 10 million patients in the United States alone, the majority of which are women. Symptoms of fibromyalgia include muscle and bone aching all over the body, physical fatigue and stiffness, insomnia, and multiple tender points in the body. Fibromyalgia can also cause psychological problems such as anxiety, depression, memory loss, and difficulty in concentrating. Researchers at Tufts University Medical Center conducted a study on the therapeutic value of Taijiquan in patients with fibromyalgia, following the rules of modern randomized clinical trial research. They divided 66 fibromyalgia patients into a "Taijiquan group" and a "fitness class". The "Taijiquan group" practiced Taijiquan twice a week, 1 hour each time, for 12 consecutive weeks. "Fitness class" participated in fitness class exercise twice a week, with mild stretching warm-up training before exercising. At the end of the 12-week trial, the researchers administered the Fibromyalgia Physical and Psychological Improvement Questionnaire. The results showed that compared with the "fitness class", the participants in the "Taijiquan group" scored higher and their symptoms improved significantly. Measures of the improvement included: reduced pain; improved ability to perform daily activities without pain; significantly less fatigue, depression, and anxiety; and better overall quality of life. The results of the study showed that practicing Taijiquan can effectively relieve muscle pain, and improve the sleep quality and physical fitness of the patients. What's more, the benefits of Taijiquan still persisted for the patient's follow-up visit up to 24 weeks.

These findings were published in the August 19, 2010 issue of the New England Journal of Medicine. Taijiquan is featured in one of the highest-level medical journals in the medical world. Two years later, another major Taijiquan study was grandly launched. This time it was for Parkinson's patients.

Patients with Parkinson's disease, their balance is severely impaired, resulting in decreased functional ability and increased risk of falling. Researchers at the Oregon Research Institute conducted a randomized controlled trial to investigate if a tailored Taijiquan program could improve postural control in people with idiopathic Parkinson's disease. 195 Parkinson's disease patients with stage 1 to 4 disease on the Hoehn and Yahr staging scale (which ranges from 1 to 5, with higher stages indicating more severe disease) were randomly assigned to the Taijiquan practice group, resistance training group, and stretching group. Patients participated in two 60-minute exercise sessions per week for 24 weeks. The researchers measured changes from baseline in the limits-of-stability test (maximum excursion and directional control; range from 0 to 100%), gait and strength, scores on functional-reach and timed up-and-go tests, motor scores on the Unified Parkinson's Disease Rating Scale, and a number of falls.

The Taijiquan protocol consisted of six movements integrated into an eight-form routine. For the goal of maintaining balance through postural control, the protocol was specifically designed to tax balance and gait by having participants perform symmetric and diagonal movements, such as weight shifting, controlled displacement of the center of mass over the base of support, ankle sways, and anterior–posterior and lateral stepping. Natural breathing was integrated into the Taijiquan sessions. The results showed that the maximal exercise performance of the Taijiquan group was consistently better than that of the resistance training and stretching groups. The study also showed that the Taijiquan group performed better than the resistance training group in terms of stride length and functional reach. Compared with the stretching group, Taijiquan reduced the incidence of falls. The effect of Taijiquan training was maintained at 3 months after the intervention. Taijiquan training reduces balance impairment in people with mild to moderate Parkinson's disease, with the additional benefit of improved functional capacity and reduced falls.

These findings were published in the February 9, 2012 issue of the New England Journal of Medicine. Taijiquan once again reached the top.

Every time I read such a study, I can't help but think of Mr. He Ming. This may constitute a collective commemoration for Mr. He Ming that is not only mine but can？？

人生过半，学习过不同的专业和技能，受到很多名师的指点。

数点这些名师似乎给人一种炫耀自己的印象。其实不然。我认为更多的是表达一种对于这些名师的敬仰，随着时间的流逝，这种感情还愈加强烈。甚至每一次认真地数点他们，对自己都是一种鞭策和鼓励。在山东大学从事数学学习和教学的十年，聆听过山大和前来山大讲课的多位院士的课。后来进入经济学领域，特别是在明尼苏达大学学习经济学期间，更是聆听过那么多位后来获得诺贝尔经济学奖的名师的讲课。再后来进入针灸教育，那更是与数不清的国医大师，针灸名家有着更为近距离或者视频往来。在这一篇回忆文章里，我回忆的不是我的数学院士老师们，也不是我的诺贝尔经济学奖教授们，也不是那些国医大师们，而是一个对我的太极拳，或者更广泛地说对我的健身运动产生了绝对影响的一个人，那就是何明老先生。认识了何老先生不但让我把太极拳只是一个概念变成了活灵活现的健身练习，而且还知道了易筋经、六字诀、五禽戏等各种健身气功，从此开始知道这些健身气功的价值。

　　第一次见到何老先生是在 1995 年。何老先生的女儿何新蓉大夫决定留在美国和我在美国一起发展中医后，何老先生也来美国访问。一见到何老先生，他就给我留下了铭记于生的印象。清瘦的面孔，和蔼而充满智慧，慈祥而饱经沧桑。八十五岁老人，腰板笔挺，耳聪目明，走路轻盈，思维敏捷。何老先生早年黄埔军校毕业更让我敬慕十分。中华民国和人民共和国的经历让何老先生饱经风雨沧桑也获得了那一代人特有的智慧与丰富的思想。老人一生与太极拳为伴，在重庆带出了一批又一批的学生。六十七年的太极拳教学生涯，近两万学生从中受益。老人来到美国，也把太极拳带来了。

　　那是我永远不会忘记的一幕。1995 年我们建立的中医健康中心的第一个诊所坐落在明尼苏达大学邻近的大学技术中心办公楼里。这个办公楼的活动中心大厅坐落在楼的一层正中间，有两层楼高，华灯高悬，大厅的东西两侧可以透过窗户玻璃看到外面的天空和繁星。这个大厅可以容纳 200 人开会，但是打太极拳只能容纳 50 人。大厅的一侧（北侧）有高出地面的主席台。这个主席台的设置从东到西，跨越整个大厅。每个星期三晚上，音乐响起，何老先生身穿麻素白色的宽松太极拳服，何新蓉大夫身穿浅粉红的真丝太极拳服，何老先生和何大夫在主席台上优雅地演示着"白鹤亮翅"、"野马分鬃"、"金鸡独立"，40多个学生跟随着何老先生和何大夫的潇洒自如的动作全神贯注地学习。《亚美时报》专门派记者S.A.Lucas多次来到太极拳班上采访何老先生。

何老先生只会说一些英语单词，不能用英语流畅地和美国学生进行语言交流，但是这似乎丝毫没有成为他们之间的沟通障碍。每次太极拳课后，一些学生总是围着他询问问题，他们之间就像没有任何语言障碍一样。另外他还有一个绝招，只要他感觉学生们的问题是太极拳方面的，他就用太极拳的演示做出回答。何老先生把太极拳的动作和各种姿势变成了世界通用语言。多么可爱的老人啊！

何伯伯曾经在我家住过几次。每次住在我家，太阳升起的时候，何老先生在我家后院里增加了一道风景。我家的后院被茂密的一片树林遮掩着。几十年的枫树、橡树、铁树、杨树高纵入云。每天早晨就在太阳穿过树林从东边斜照进我家后院里的时候，何伯伯已经开始打起他的太极拳了。碧绿的草坪上矫健的老人已经在做"手挥琵琶"、"搂膝拗步"、"双峰贯耳"了。周围树上的鸟叫就是伴随着何伯伯太极拳姿的音乐。这些优美的动中有静、静中有动的姿势完全融化到自然中去了。

每天早晨打完太极拳后，何伯伯就坐下来记他的笔记。他的笔记本上记满了各方面的信息。我们讨论的有趣的事情他都记录下来。还有一些中文报纸《世界日报》、《星岛日报》上的报道，他剪下来贴在自己的笔记本上。

在我家居住的日子里，他还天天都在抄写《菜根谭》。也正好是他在一边抄写《菜根谭》、一边吟诵那些名句的时候，我对"无事宜寂寂，有事宜惺惺"、"心无物欲，即是秋空霁海；坐有琴书，便成石室丹丘"、"闲中不放过，忙中有受用；静中不落空，动中有受用；暗中不欺隐，明中有受用"、"人情世态，不宜认真"的理解更加深刻了。一位赢得无穷尊敬的老人，他本身就是这些警世通言的化身。

自我按摩是我们太极拳课中的加餐。静坐安神、意守丹田，自我按摩足三里、三阴交、内关正是这些加餐里的名吃。指压安眠穴、点压太冲穴、合谷穴是这些加餐里的调料。难以计数的病人和学生们从这些带有东方智慧的保健活动中受益无穷。

我曾带何老先生和家人们去明尼苏达大学植物园，他对那里的花草、树木、小溪、池塘表现出极大的兴趣。椴树、枫树、蜡树、槐树依地势成林，此起彼伏。在山楂树、海棠树林相间的草地上，老人带着我们打起了太极拳。我们的举动不但吸引了一些游园的人，而且周围的松鼠都直立起来望着我们。何老先生打完一个短式的太极拳后说道，"你们看，松鼠也想打太极拳了！"

何老先生几次来明尼苏达，对明尼苏达留下了深刻的美好印象。1999年，我们一起专程到纽约参观，因为人多，我们住在了一个上海人开的家庭旅馆。房东对纽约的盛赞如同对老家上海一样。六十多岁的房东极其得意地赞扬道，纽约是一个极具刺激性的城市，自由女神，灯红酒绿，车水马龙，昼夜不停，在这里不会得老年痴呆症的。她比喻纽约就如同一块臭豆腐，闻着臭，吃着香。何伯伯立刻回答道，我们明尼苏达有北美最大的苏比利湖，明州就像一个白面馒头，看着香，闻着更香，越嚼越香，越嚼越有味道。大家哈哈大笑。老人反应之快令人惊艳，反应之敏锐令人称赞，幽默的回答也表达了对明尼苏达的深厚感情。

一九九九年美国中医学院正式开学。何新蓉大夫是太极拳课的任课老师。何明伯伯再次从重庆赶来助阵。实际上太极拳班里的很多学员并不是我们中医学院的学生，而是我们诊所的病人或者病人介绍过来的家人和朋友。太极拳课和气功课是中医学院所有课程中仅有的向公众和社区开放的课程。很多太极拳课的学员也是奔着何老先生来的。有从芝加哥、加拿大边境开车七-八个小时赶来上课的。他从1995年到1999年多次来美开展太极拳健身讲学，积累了很多追随者和粉丝，因此一听说何老先生继续参加带课，大家都来复习，这样太极拳班特别大，我们的课继续在大楼的活动中心举行。

何老先生对我们刚刚开业的中医学院给予极大的热情。那时古励大夫也刚刚离开洛杉矶来到明尼苏达和我们一起发展中医。何老先生不但继续参加教授我们的太极拳课，而且也帮助我们折叠宣传广告，贴上邮票。一个老人的满怀热情有他专门留下的诗句为证：

桃园颂

一九九九年三月十日

昔日桃园义千古，今日桃园贯古今。
刘巩友爱胜皇叔，古何情义超飞云。
心想事成明灯亮，三家奋斗一个心。
六君振臂助擂鼓，不扬世界鼓不停。

万万没有想到的是，当何老先生留下这些热情的诗句时，已经离他的生命终点只有六个多月了。1999年10月28日，何伯伯永远地离我们而去了。他走得那么安详、那么平静，没有给儿女带来负担，自己也没有任何痛苦。他的那种乐观精神、好学精神留给了我们。他留给我们的太极拳我们继续着，直到今天，还将继续到永远。每隔一段时间，我总是想起那位慈祥的老人。在何伯伯逝世十周年之际，我写诗纪念：

何伯伯逝世十周年缅怀
二〇〇九年十月
万木萧疏湖氤氲，孤鸿盘旋始南巡。
幕幕陈迹立残阳，岁岁秋雨忆老人。

时光流年十春秋，正直刚毅精神存。
太极往事嘱托在，报答平生留寸心。

转眼二十年过去了，2019年10月，我们的中医学院不但建立起了针灸硕士、中医硕士，而且还建立了中医博士三个项目。在这一时间关口，又想起亲手教过我，并且给予我极大精神鼓励的何伯伯。思念之余，再次留诗表达思念之情：

何伯伯逝世二十周年缅怀
二〇一九年十月
碧水蓝天枫叶红，雁叫回荡满天空。
夜半月行向西斜，秋思无言怕恐惊。
嘉陵江畔英灵在，密西西比河边梦。
太极学子勿忘恩，往事如烟于生情。

这些小诗只是我自己对何老先生的一点纪念。谈到纪念，岂止是我自己的纪念。二十多年前，当何老先生把太极拳带到美国来的时候，太极拳还谈不上是一种医疗治疗手段。就在太极拳获得广泛传播之后，美国的医学院、医学中心开始把太极拳推到了医学殿堂里了。这可能是对何伯伯的在天之灵的最大的告慰。何老先生留下的诗篇，我的纪念诗都与两本医学杂志保留在一起了。这两本医学杂志是 2010 年和 2012 年的两期《新英格兰医学杂志》。在这两起医学杂志上刊登着美国科学家们进行的两项太极拳临床随机对照实验。这两项研究分别是对肌纤维疼痛综合症和帕金森病患者的。

肌纤维疼痛综合症是一种仅美国就有患者 1000 万患者的常见病症，大部分患者是女性。肌纤维疼痛综合症的症状包括：全身肌肉和骨骼疼痛、身体疲劳及僵硬、失眠、全身还有多处特定部位的压痛点。肌纤维疼痛综合症还会导致焦虑、抑郁、记忆力减退和注意力不集中等心理问题。美国塔夫斯大学医学中心的研究人员对太极拳治疗肌纤维疼痛患者进行了按照现代临床试验设计要求的研究。他们将 66 名纤维性肌痛患者分成了"太极拳组"和"健身班组"。"太极拳组"每周练太极拳两次，每次 1 小时，连续 12 周。"健身班组"每周参加两次健身班锻炼，锻炼前有轻度拉伸的热身训练。为期 12 周的实验结束后，研究者们进行"纤维性肌痛身体和心理症状改善情况问卷调查"。调查结果显示，相对于"健身班组"，"太极拳组"

参加者得分更高，症状明显改善。改善的指标包括：疼痛减少；不受疼痛困扰而进行日常活动的能力提高；疲劳、抑郁和焦虑明显更少；总体生活质量更高。研究结果显示练太极拳能有效缓解肌肉痛，患者的睡眠质量和体质也得到相当的改善。更为甚者，对于病人的延续到 24 周的追踪访问，练太极拳的这些好处还仍然存在。

这项研究成果发表在 2010 年 8 月 19 日出版的《新英格兰医学杂志》上。太极拳登上了医学界最高级别的医学杂志上。两年之后，又有一项重磅太极拳研究隆重推出。这一次是针对帕金森病患者。

对于帕金森病患者，他们的平衡能力严重受损，由此导致功能能力下降和跌倒风险增加。俄勒冈研究院的研究人员进行了一项随机对照试验，他们用量身定制的太极拳计划研究是否可以改善特发性帕金森病患者的姿势控制。195 名患有 1 至 4 期的帕金森病患者随机分配到太极拳组、阻力训练组或伸展运动组。患者每周参加两次 60 分钟的锻炼，实验持续 24 周。研究人员测量稳定性极限测试中相对于基线的变化以及步态和力量的测量、功能范围和定时启动测试的得分、统一帕金森病评定量表的运动得分和跌倒次数。量身定制的太极拳包含八式招法，集中于重量平移，有支撑的重心控制位移，关节运动，前端至后端和侧身的运动，这些运动再加入了自然呼吸方法。实验结果表明太极拳组的最大运动表现始于优于阻力训练组和拉伸组。实验结果表明太极拳组在步幅和功能范围方面优于阻力训练组。与拉伸相比，太极拳降低了跌倒的发生率。太极拳训练的效果维持在 3 个月之后。这项研究太极拳训练可以减少轻度至中度帕金森病患者的平衡障碍，并且具有提高功能能力和减少跌倒的额外好处。

这项研究成果发表在 2012 年 2 月 9 日出版的《新英格兰医学杂志》上。太极拳再次登顶。

我每次读到这样的研究，不由地想起何老先生。这不就是对老人家的一种集体纪念吗！

100. "The Happy Master" of Taijiquan
太极拳的 "乐行僧"

By Li Jinquan Professor 教授

Uncle He Ming was such a happy old man. Now that we are old, we miss Uncle He even more. He was an easy-going, kind-hearted handsome man who laughed often, lived a simple life, and was psychologically satisfied. He taught Taijiquan with all his might, was very patient, neither fast nor slow, taught students repeatedly, and never took advantage of his seniority to scold others. I said that he was a "happy guru". He crossed the sea to the northern kingdom of the New World, hoping that our younger generation could maintain a strong energy, qi and spirit no matter how busy life got.

At the turn of the century, Uncle He traveled from Sichuan to Minnesota to visit his daughter Xinrong He, a doctor of traditional Chinese medicine, so that we had the opportunity to meet him. Every Sunday morning, he volunteered to teach us Taijiquan in the park through personal example as well as verbal instruction, which was very moving. He studied at the Whampoa Military Academy when he was young and even won the school's Taijiquan championship. He has practiced Taijiquan all his life without interruption. He said that the long-distance train on the mainland was very slow, and the stop time was very long, so he got off the train and played Taijiquan on the platform, which attracted a lot of attention. When we first met him, Uncle He was already eighty years old, but he was agile and had great strength. Occasionally, Uncle He would demonstrate a move, and with a slight push and to our great astonishment, the much younger student was forced several steps backwards!

As the saying goes: "The master shows you the way, but you have to take the first step." In the first few years, I insisted on practicing Taijiquan. Although my movements were clumsy, I always felt comfortable in my body and mind after finishing Taijiquan. Later, for some reason, I began to be lazy, and gradually stopped practicing. When I thought about it, I felt ashamed and indebted to Uncle He's painstaking efforts in teaching Taijiquan. However, some of the things he taught have also been integrated into my life, such as abdominal breathing when I am stressed, and thinking of the slowness of Taijiquan when I am anxious.

A smart and diligent student learned the true meaning of Taijiquan from Uncle He. For a while, he returned to Taichung to take care of his centenarian mother. He went to Taichung Park to practice Taijiquan every morning. The morning exercisers saw his beautiful postures and wanted to learn from him. Like Uncle He, he started free Taijiquan classes and practiced together every morning for a year. After my friend returned to the United States, the Taijiquan class that was developed in Taichung Park is still actively continuing. "Inadvertently sowing seeds led to great big trees", and if Uncle He knew his legacy was spread around the world, he would definitely be happy forever.

Uncle He taught us not only Tai Chi, but also how to be a human being. His calligraphy was excellent, and he often wrote banners encouraging us to practice Taijiquan. What I remember are the three words "Jing, Qi, Shen".

When I chat with him sometimes, he mentioned the War of Resistance Against Japanese Aggression and suddenly burst into tears, which was deeply touching. During the civil war between the Kuomintang and the Communist Party, he stayed in the Chengdu headquarters of the Whampoa Military Academy as an instructor.

Fortunately, he was not overthrown by the turbulence of the times. Because he was so nice and kind to people there were many who stood to protect him.

With such a good father, Dr. He Xinrong is also kind in nature, has friends all over the world, and takes care of patients with special dedication. It is our pleasure to recognize these two individuals.

何明伯伯是最乐天知命的老人。我们自己初老了，更常常怀念何伯伯。他平易亲切，笑口常开，生活简单，心理满足，真潇洒。他倾囊相授太极拳，非常有耐心，不慌不急，一遍一遍教，也从不倚老卖老，从不教训人。我说他是"乐行僧"，渡海到新大陆的北国，就是希望我们晚辈在忙碌的工作之余能够保持旺盛的精、气、神。

何伯伯在世纪之交从四川到明尼苏达，探视中医生女儿何新蓉大夫，我们才有机会和他结缘。每周日清晨，他自愿在公园教我们太极拳，融合言教身教，感人至深。他年轻时就读於黄埔军校，得过全校太极拳比赛冠军。他一辈子打拳，毫不间断。他说当年大陆的长途火车很慢，中途停站的时间很长，他就下车在月台上打太极拳，吸引許多目光。我们初识他的时候，何伯伯已八七高龄，但身手矫健，力气很大，偶尔做个示范动作，轻轻一弹，五十多岁的学友就退了好几步，让我们啧啧称奇。

俗話说："师傅領进门，修行在自己。"我有几年还不忘打太极拳，虽然动作笨拙，总觉得打完拳以后身心舒泰。后来不知什么原因，开始疏懒，渐渐就荒费了，想起来就觉得惭愧，辜负了何伯伯传法的苦心。不过他传教的一些东西也融入了生活中，例如压力大的时候做腹式呼吸，心理着急时就想到太极拳慢的道理。

有位聪明而勤奋的学友从何伯伯那里学到了太极拳的真谛。有一阵子，他回到台中照顾百岁老母，每天早上到台中公园打太极拳，晨运的人看到姿势优美，想跟他学。他像何伯伯一样，免费开班，每天早上一起练习，达一年之久。我的朋友回美国以后，那个太极拳班在台中公园开拓，自主的生命，继续不辍。何伯伯的遗泽在异地散播，无心插柳柳成阴，他若地下有知，一定会大笑三声。

何伯伯教我们的不仅是太极拳，还有做人。他的书法极好，还写条幅送我们，我得到的是"精气神"三个字。我有时找他聊天，他提起抗日战争突然老泪纵横，令人动容。国共易帜，他留在黄埔军校成都本部当教官，幸未被时代的乱流打翻，因为他厚道，对人好，自称保护他的人很多。

有这么好的父亲，何新蓉大夫也是秉性善良，广结善缘，照顾病人特别尽心尽力。认得这一对父女，是我们的福气。

101. My Memories of Taiji Master He, Ming
我对太极拳大师何明的回忆

By **Cary Hakam, DAOM, L.Ac.** 中医博士

I first met Master He in 1998. I had been working as an interpreter and secretary for his daughter, Dr. He, Xinrong, for about a year at the TCM Health Center in Dinkytown. He was of a slight build and sported a permanent, infectious smile. I remember straining to understand his thick Sichuan accent when he first joined his daughter in teaching the Yang-style Taiji class at the American Academy of Acupuncture and Oriental Medicine (AAAOM). Since I was the interpreter for the class, I also was called to help demonstrate the martial application of the movements. Feigning the aggressor, I would lunge at Master He, only to find myself flung across the floor, or swung off my feet by this petite man, almost three times my age. Try as I might, I could not budge him from his grounded stance. Laughing, he would demonstrate to the class the power of centering and using one's waist to lead the movements of defensive blocks, or attacking strikes. How could an 87-year-old man throw me, a physically fit 33-year-old, around the room as if I were nothing but a stuffed doll? Instantaneously, Master He changed my opinion of Taiji, from one of curious interloper to that of awestruck believer.

In the few months that I was lucky enough to be in the company of Master He, I saw how he demonstrated the way of Taiji in how he carried himself in his actions and the way he emanated this philosophy throughout his life. I was fortunate to hear many stories of Master He's life while working next to Dr. Xinrong He. She often teaches her patients how to live a healthy, virtuous life through storytelling, and invariably, many of these stories were about her father.

I went on to study Taiji, and co-teach with Dr. Xinrong He each trimester at AAAOM for the next twenty-odd years. Master He's influence never left me all these years and I still recall the humbling power of the "old master". There is a word/character in Chinese: De (德)which translates to something like, virtue-power, though it also means much more. When I think of this character, 德 , my mind goes right to Master He Ming.

我第一次见到何明大师是在 1998 年。我在 Dinkytown 中医保健中心为他的女儿何新蓉博士做了大约一年的翻译和秘书。何明大师身材瘦小,露出着永久、富有感染力的微笑。我记得,当他第一次和女儿一起在美国针灸与东方医学学院 (AAAOM) 教授杨式太极拳课时,我正在努力理解他浓重的四川口音。因为我是这个班的翻译,所以我也被叫来协助演示武术应用的动作。我假装是侵略者,向他冲去,却发现自己被这个年纪几乎是我三倍的小个子男人扔在地板上了,或是被他甩到地上。尽管我尽力努力,但我还是无法回避他的还击,从他那脚踏实地的位置上挪开。他会笑着向班级展示定力和用腰的力量来引导防守的动作,或进攻的动作。一个 87 岁的男人怎么能把我,一个 33 岁的人,扔到房间里,好像我只是一个充气娃娃?他立刻改变了我对太极拳的看法,从一个好奇的迷茫者变成了一个忠实的信徒。

在我有幸和何大师在一起的几个月里,我看到了他如何展示太极拳的方式,如何在行动中表现自己,以及他如何在他的一生中宣扬太极拳哲学。在和何新蓉博士一起工作的时候,我有幸听到了许多关于何大师生平的故事。她经常通过讲故事来帮助她的病人如何过健康、高尚的生活,而这些故事中有很多都是有关于她父亲的。

我继续学习太极拳，在接下来的二十多年里，每隔三个月我与何新蓉博士在 AAAOM 共同教学。这些年来，我仍然记得这位何明大师的美德的力量，他的影响力多年来从未离开过我。我还记得"老拳师"的谦卑的力量。中文中有一个单词"德"，翻译为类似于美德 - 力量，但我认为它的含义远不止于此。每当我想到"德"这个字的时候，我的脑子就会想到何明大师。

102. In Memory of Mr. He Ming
追思何明老先生

Dictated by He Zhini

I am very fortunate to meet Mr. He Ming. It was 1995, when he took my hand and said that I was a girl from the He's family, just like his daughter.I was so happy I felt younger (actually,I was in my 70s at the time).

Mr. He was very kind, warm, friendly,approachable, and treated me like a family member.I felt very happy and safe when I was with him.

Mr. He is very kind and caring, because I have bad eyesight, so Mr. He specially adapted a very short course of Taiqiquan to teach me.

I was saddened when he passed away, and he was a wonderful person. So my husband and I specially invited professionals to decorate the memorial service venue, bought a lot of flowers, and held a memorial service in the backyard of Mr. He's daughter's house. About 200 of his Taijiquan students came that day, and everyone played Taijiquan in the backyard to commemorate him in this special way. I am very relieved to have done what I should have done for the old gentleman Mr. He.

我很幸运，有缘认识何明老先生。那是 1995 年，当时他拉着我的手，说我是何家姑娘，我好开心。我仿佛变的年轻了。（实际那时我已 70 多岁）他为人亲切、和蔼、热情、好有亲和力，待我如亲人一般，和他在一起，非常快乐、非常有安全感。

何老先生很善良，很有爱心，因为我眼睛不好，他特别为我编了一套很短的太极拳来教我。

后来他去世了，我很难过，他是一个很好的人。于是我和我先生特别请了专业人员来布置会场，买了许多的鲜花，在何老先生的女儿家后院开了追思会。当天他的太极拳学生来了约 200 人左右，大家在后院打太极拳，用这种特别的方式纪念他。我感到很欣慰，为何老先生做了一件应该做的事。

103. In Memory of My Father 纪念老父亲

By He Murong

It has been 23 years since my father left us, but I feel like he has never left me. His voice and smile often come to my mind. His whole life was spent caring for and helping others. His kindness and sincerity won the respect and affection of many people. He often tells us to be kind and help others. Helping others is helping ourselves. "The roses in her hand, the flavor in mine" (the meaning of this idiom is "Send people roses, hands have lingering fragrance".)

He spent his life caring for others, and take pleasure in helping others. His kindness and sincerity have won the respect and touch of many people. there were always noble people to help him, and he got through whatever bad luck and made it safely to old age. Influenced by my father, I am also willing to help others, and benefit a lot. In 1996, I went to Shanghai for a very tricky thing. While I was waiting at Suzhou station, an old lady who was trembling with a plastic bag came by me. I asked her why she came to Suzhou alone, and she replied that her daughter had passed away a long time ago, and that she visited her grave every year. I comfort her and gave her 200 Yuan as we talked. The results werealmost as if I was being rewarded for a good deed, the difficult thing was easily resolved.

My colleague's child was hospitalized and needed to borrow money. No one was willing to lend it to him. He cried in frustration. Seeing the way he was crying and running nose, I remembered what my father said:

"When others are sick, in trouble, or in difficult time, I can help as much as possible." I decided to lend him money. Some people advised me, don't lend money to him. And told me that he may not be able to pay it back. He needed more than 20 thousand Yuan. I didn't have so much cash. So I sold all my stocks to solve his urgent needs. Later, the stock market crashed sharply, but my stock had already been sold without any loss. After my colleague's son recovered, he went to college and found a stable job, and the money was paid back to me. I declined the interest which he gave me. My colleague said he would always thank me for saving his child's life!

Our He family has had many scholars since our ancestors, and the fifth ancestor was the last prime minister of the Qing Dynasty. His ancestral house became our He family ancestral hall and a key cultural relic protection unit in Anhui Province. My great-grandfather served as county magistrate three times, he was enthusiastic about public welfare, helping the poor, releasing lives, and burying his bones (the poor had no money to bury them when they died). When he returned to his hometown, he had no money to buy land.

My father inherited the great qualities of his grandfather and took pleasure in helping others. Every year when the school year starts, he sent money back to our hometown to support the children of our relatives to study. After I started working, I also followed the ways of my father by supporting the children and preventing them from dropping out of school. Education is the most important thing. Now they are all talented and established, and they have become the leaders or technical backbones of the teams they are

I have been frail and sick ever since I was a child. I have experienced gas poisoning, chlorine poisoning, ovarian tumor removal, extensive herpes zoster, a fractured thoracic spine, I had typhoid, and I also had cancer at 65. But because of how my father's strong and optimistic spirit and love for Taijiquan have influenced me, I survived and regained my health after each serious illness.

I was an associate professor at the university and was rated as an excellent teacher many times. I did not retire until was 63 years old. Then I returned to class until I was 65. Now that I am 78 years old, I can still practice Taijiquan for an hour every day, swim 1000 meters in 35 minutes, and carry forward with teaching Taijiquan and swimming, the family heirlooms that my father gave me! I will keep teaching Taijiquan and swimming! I am very proud that I have lived up to the expectations of my late father!

I'm so lucky enough to have such a good father. I want to learn from my late father for the rest of my life and pass on a healthy and optimistic outlook on life with great love in life and deeds, and become a real winner in life!

父亲离开我们已经 23 年了，感觉他永远没有离开过我。他的音容笑貌常常浮现在我的脑海里，他常常告诫我们要心怀善意，帮助他人，助人就是助己。送人玫瑰，手有余香。他的一生关心他人、助人为乐。他的善良真诚，获得了许多人的尊敬和感动。因此在他坎坷的人生中也是常有贵人相助，能逢凶化吉平安渡过。受父亲的影响，我也乐于助人，并受益匪浅。

1996 年我去上海办一件很棘手的事。在苏州车站上来一个拿着塑料口袋颤颤巍巍的老太太，我问她怎么一个人来苏州？她说我女儿去世很久了，我来给她上坟，每年我都来。我心里为她难过，我安慰她还送她 200 元。结果好心真有好报，非常难办的事竟轻松地完成了。

我的同事的孩子住院需要借钱，没人愿意借，他哭了，看见他眼泪鼻涕的样子，我想起父亲说的话"当别人有病、有灾、有难时，能帮尽量帮"，我决定借钱给他。好些人劝我不要借，说他可能还不起。

他需要两万多元。我当时也没有这么多现钱，就把股票全卖了，解决了他的燃眉之急。后来股市大跌，但是我的股票早已抛出，没有受损失。同事的儿子病好后，读了大专找了份稳定的工作，钱也还了我，我谢绝了他给我的利息。同事说他永远感谢我，救了孩子的命。

我们何氏家族从先辈起出了多名进士，更有五世祖是清朝末代宰相。他的祖屋成为我们何家祠堂，也成为安徽省重点文物保护单位。祖父虽曾任三任县官，但他热心公益，济贫，放生，埋尸（穷人死了无钱埋），当他告老还乡时，却没有钱买地。我的父亲传承了祖父的优秀品质，助人为乐。每到逢年开学就寄钱回老家，支持亲戚家的孩子们读书，我工作后也学老父亲一块寄钱，不让亲戚家的孩子们失学，教育为大。后来他们长大工作了，都很有才能，很有实力，成为所在团队的领导者或技术骨干。

我从小体弱多病，经历过煤气中毒，氯气中毒，卵巢肿瘤切除，大面积带状疱疹，胸椎骨折，还得过伤寒，65岁还患过癌症。由于老父亲坚强乐观的精神和热爱太极拳运动影响了我，每次大病后我都能够健康地活了下来。还在大学里任副教授，多次评为优秀教师，工作到63岁才退休。后来又返聘上课到65岁。现在我已经78岁了，依然能够坚持每天练太极拳一小时，游泳1000米/35分钟，还能将父亲给我的传家宝—太极拳与游泳发扬光大，坚持教他人太极拳和游泳！感到很骄傲，没有辜负老父亲的期望培养！

我很幸运，有这样的好父亲。我要一辈子学习老父亲，对生命充满热爱，保持乐观的人生态度，并传承下去，成为人生真正的赢家！

104. Deep Memory 深深的怀念

By He Shiyuan

My father was strict with me. Ever since I was a child, I was told that one should love his country and value friendship. Moreover, I was asked to practice calligraphy and Taijiquan. In fact, my father himself taught me these skills and practiced together with me.

He also took me to travel around the beautiful rivers and mountains to learn more about our motherland.

Carefully nurtured by my father for decades, it was not until I grew up that I began to understand his love and efforts in raising me . Now, I am already 76 years old. I can still enjoy mountain climbing, Gliding at high altitude. Paint mountains and rivers with a brush in hand and have a sincere heart for the motherland, all of which come from the health, wisdom and love that my father painstakingly passed on to me. When I was 65, I still got my plane pilot license with great confidence.

There is one thing that I keep in my deep heart.

It was in the 1990s when my father returned from abroad to see me. At that time, I was in Jiangshan, Quzhou City, Zhejiang Province, conducting a research on the Japanese envoys' way to China by land and sea in the Tang Dynasty. After picking him up, I accompanied him to climb the Mount Jianglang, get through the Xianxia Pass and visit the Qinghe ancient street. The old man ascended the mountain and crossed the river at such a brisk pace that no one would believe he was already in his eighties.

At the foot of the Mount Jianglang, we paid a visit to the Museum of the War of Chinese People's Resistance against Japanese Aggression which was under construction. In the old dwellings, my father burst into tears at the sight of the veterans' stuff. He and many of these veterans were alumni of Whampoa Military Academy. Seeing the photos and relics, the old man's memory went back to the past of studying at Whampoa Military Academy and the anti-Japanese battles in Wuhan, Zhejiang and Fujian.

Standing on the Xianxia Pass, where the 49th Army had killed the Japanese invader Colonel Kameta in the Zhejiang-Fujian battle, my father couldn't help singing out loud the poem *Man Jiang Hong*("*The River All Red*") by Yuefei , a national hero in the Southern Song Dynasty, which encouraged them to go to the front line. "Wrath sets on end my hair; I lean on railings where I see the drizzling rain has ceased."

During the visit to Jiangshan City, from those county sages in Quzhou, he heard about Zhu Yunzhe, the friend of Yue Fei and how he risked his life to rescue Yuefei. My father was so deeply moved that he told me I should conduct a thorough research on the matter and report to him. After his departure, I started my hard work on it.

Zhu Yunzhe, a resident of the Mount Jianglang, was a scholar in 1100, and close friend of Yue Fei. His father, Zhu Chen, minister of the Military Defence advocated fight against alien attack and once strongly recommended Yue Fei to the Emperor.

In 1141, Yue Fei was put into prison by Qin Hui (chief minister in the Southern Song Dynasty who advocated surrender to alien attack) while Zhu Yunzhe was fighting together with General Han Shizhong at the front line. After he got the news, he risked his life and submitted a memorial to the Emperor: "I am willing to vouch for Yue Fei with the lives of more than 70 family members of my own. Please release him."

Hearing that Yue Fei was in danger, he hurried back from the front. On his way to Fuyang, Hangzhou, he heard that Yue Fei and his son had been executed. Wearied and worried, he passed away abruptly and was buried in the Mount Baisheng in Fuyang.

Following the instruction of my father, I have been to Jiangshan and Fuyang many times, but couldn't get any detailed information. Later, with the help of my friend Xu Deqin, I finally got a chance to see the precious genealogy of Zhu's family in Jiangshan. As for the Mount Baisheng and Baisheng County in Fuyang where Zhu Yunzhe had been buried, I have also visited numerous times only to find there are no longer such names.

In a-thousand-year-carefully-preserved Zhu's genealogy, I found out a very important thing, that is the origination and proceeding of Yue Fei's famous poem *Man Jiang Hong*.

It turned out that after the great victory in Zhuxian Town, Yue Fei wrote a poem *Man Jiang Hong* to Zhu Yunzhe. Then Yunzhe wrote back to him for a reply. Inspired by Yunzhe's words,Yue fei wrote another new one, that is the well-known patriotic poem in which we find those very familiar lines as "When we've reconquered our lost land, in triumph would return our army grand."

In the poem, such words as "breaking through Helan Mountain" and "in triumph would return our army grand" were derived from Zhu Yunzhe's poem. In Zhu's genealogy, there are three poems of *Man Jiang Hong* we found, that is Yue Fei's original one, Zhu Yongzhe's one for reply and Yue Fei's final *Man Jiang Hong*. The genealogy recorded in detail the deep friendship between Zhu and Yue, which is very precious.

As for the Mount Baisheng, it is not until many years later that I inquired into the Fuyang County annals during the reign of Kangxi (1662-1722). It reads that "the Mount Baisheng, 30 miles north of the county, was a famous Taoist mountain, which enjoys the beautiful scenery with eighteen ancient post stations...". Later through the on-site investigation, I found that the Mount Baisheng is now known as the Mount Xiyan. The road at the foot of mountain was an important post road from north and south to Lin'an (The capital city of the Southern Song Dynasty). Some famous poets in the Tang Dynasty such as Bai Juyi and Liu Yuxi had written poems singing the praise of this mountain.

It took me around ten years that followed my father's instructions and found out the truth. Unfortunately, in 1999, my father died of illness in Minnesota, USA.

Last September, I went to Fuyang again and finally climbed up the Mount Baisheng.

Known as the Mount Xiyan now, the Mount Baisheng was said to be the place where Ge Hong (a famous Taoist, 282-363) made the pills of immortality and became an immortal in the daytime. The Chinese characters Baisheng just mean becoming an immortal in the daytime. And the county at the foot of the mountain is called Baisheng County. Due to its unique scenery, many celebrities paid their visits to the mountain in the Tang Dynasty, and in the Ming Dynasty, it was renamed to the Mount Xiyan. At the foot of the mountain, there was an ancient post road to Bianjin (the capital city of the Northern Song Dynasty). Today, the Mount Xiyan belongs to Yinhu Sub-district, Fuyang District and is keeping developed.

Unfortunately, the tomb of Zhu Yunzhe could not be found and may no longer exist. But as long as the towering green mountain is standing still there, the righteous spirit of Yunzhe will always remain in my heart.

I still remember that many years ago when my father left Jiangshan, he said to me, "One must be loyal to his country and be true to his friends. This is the spirit of Yunzhe and we should keep it in mind forever..."

Though the bones of national heroes were buried in the green mountains of Fuyang, their loyalty to the country has been handed down for hundreds of generations.

Never shall I forget the loving-kindness and principles of righteousness that my father left with me.

父亲对我严格。自小要我练字，打太极拳，要我重义爱国。而且他身教力行，带我练字，教我太极拳，陪我山川读华夏，荫恩数十载。

直到我长大成人，才深知父亲的胸襟，深知父亲育儿之苦心。今朝我已 76 岁，还能体能纵越险岭，高空滑翔，手能挥笔写山河，思能辩古爱华夏。在我 65 岁时还信心满满的考取了飞机驾驶执照。这全靠父亲苦心传给我的健康、智慧和爱心…。

有一件事，我深记于心。

那是上世纪九十年代。那年，父亲归国看我。其时我正在衢州江山，研究日本遣唐史空海求学之路。接到父亲后，我陪老人爬江郎山，游仙霞关，访清河古街。老人登山入水健步如飞，谁也看不出已是八十多岁老翁。

在江郎山下，我们去拜访了修建中的抗战纪念馆。在古拙的山居，见到许多抗战老兵的故物时，父亲沧然泪下。这些老兵中许多是老父黄埔的校友，看到照片和故物，老人又想起了当年黄埔军校求学和武汉会战、浙闽会战的往事…。

在浙闽会战中，49 军击毙日寇龟田大佐的仙霞岭上，父亲不禁唱起了当年激励他们上前线的岳飞《满江红》。"怒发冲冠凭栏处，潇潇雨歇…"

在江山市访问时，他听衢州乡贤讲说了抗虏英雄岳飞的好友，祝允哲舍身救飞的事迹，他深为感动。嘱我一定要细细调研此事，并详告之。父亲离浙后，我就开始了艰苦的考证。

祝允哲，江郎峰下人，宋元符三年进士，为岳飞抗金的挚友。其父祝臣，主战派，官至上柱国兵部尚书。曾向徽宗力荐岳飞，为岳飞的伯乐。

绍兴十一年（即 1411 年），岳飞为秦桧所陷下狱。祝永哲时与韩世忠正在前线。闻飞受陷后，冒死向皇帝上疏："愿以全家 70 余口担保，岳忠，请释"。后闻岳飞事险，急从前线返朝。在杭州富阳途中，忽闻岳飞父子已经遇害，劳顿心急，顿时身亡。后葬于富阳白升山。

为尊父嘱，我曾多次奔走于江山和富阳两地。但未得详解。后在好友徐德勤帮助下，终于见到了珍贵的江郎山祝氏家谱。而永哲安葬的富阳白升乡白升山，踏访多次，早已无留此山此乡名。

在珍藏千年祝氏家谱中，我看到了一件特别重要的大事。岳飞名词《满江红》的序进。

原来朱仙镇大胜后，岳飞写了满江红词赠祝允哲。允哲也即回填满江红一首相赠。岳在祝的回词中得到启发，重写新词。此新词即我们耳熟能详的"待收拾旧山河，朝天阙…"名传千古的爱国诗词《满江红》。

其中"踏破贺兰山缺"，"朝天阙"等词句即源于祝允哲词。家谱中，收有《满江红》三首；岳飞原词，祝永哲回词和岳飞《满江红》后词。字谱详载祝岳情深，甚为珍贵。

而白升山，直到多年后，我才查到康熙富阳县志，"白升山，在县北三十里，为道教名山，山绝秀丽，有故驿十八景……"。后我经实地勘证，白升山即今西岩山。山下之路即宋代南北进京临安的重要驿道…。

白居易、刘禹锡等皆有诗颂赞此山。我尊父嘱，查明此事，前后十年。

可惜，父亲已于 1999 年病逝于美国明尼苏达。

去年九月，我赶赴富阳探访，终于登上了白升山。

白升山又名西岩山，传葛洪在此练丹，曾白日升仙，故名白升山。山下之乡亦名白升乡，唐代因此山有奇绝西岩，名士多访之，明代改名西岩山。山脚至今遗有通京古驿道。今西岩山属富阳银湖街道，正在开发中。

可惜，允哲墓地遍踏青山，于未找到，也许己不复存在。但巍巍青山犹在，允哲大义永存我心…。

　　我想起了多年前老父临离江山时曾告我："于国忠，于友义，此，允哲之精神。吾辈当牢记之…。"富阳青山埋忠骨，爱国大义百代传…。

　　父亲留给我们的恩与义当永记于心。

105. The Most Precious Wealth My Father Left 父亲留下的最宝贵的财富

By Dr. He Xingrong

In the 1930s, my father suffered from tuberculosis and hemoptysis (there was no cure for this disease at the time). My father was introduced to learn Taijiquan by Zeng Shouchang, director of the Shaoxing National Martial Arts Museum. He practices Taijiquan every day. Practice Taijiquan actually cured his tuberculosis without medicine.

Since then, he began to be a volunteer to teach Taijiquan for 67 years. He hoped that everyone all over the world would know how to practice Taijiquan and enjoy the good life brought by Taijiquan. Father said this is his lifelong ideal and responsibility! My father was a Taijiquan sower. There are his students all over Chongqing, Beijing, and Guangzhou city. Not only that, father also spread the flower of Taijiquan to the United States. Many American students even drive seven to eight hours to learn from him.

From youth to old, my father never stopped teaching Taijiquan. He said that whenever he is alive, he'll never stop teaching Taijiquan untill he goes to see The God.

This persistence, this kind of great love, let us, deeply educated!

Since then, he began to be a volunteer to teach Taijiquan for 67 years. He hoped that everyone all over the world would know how to practice Taijiquan and enjoy the good life brought by Taijiquan. Father said this is his lifelong ideal and responsibility! My father was a Taijiquan sower. There are his students all over Chongqing, Beijing, Nanjing, and Shenzhen city. Not only that, father also spread the flower of Taijiquan to the United States. Many American students even drive seven to eight hours to learn from him.

Father taught us to cultivate morality before practicing martial arts. Taijiquan is a kind of civilized boxing with cultural He warned us: kindness, optimism, tolerance, perseverance, diligenec, studiousness; sincerity, respect for teachers and love for friends, benevolence, and righteousness are the spirit of Taijiquan.

Father also asked us forever away from alcohol, sex and wealth, angry wine, women, avarice and temper-- the four cardinal vices. Learn to be grateful. In China, we say   a "drop of water given in need return a burst of spring in deed". Every day he kept a diary to check what he did wrong? Have done reading and practicing writing, His words and deeds, always inspire us. even His hearty laugh, deeply engraved in our minds also. All three brothers and sisters have also developed the habit of laughter.

There are two small things that I will never forget:

1.   While my father and I were waiting for a trolleybus, a man came to ask the way. My father told him It is not far away, and he can go there without waiting for the bus. So the man went away. Then I noticed that the man's legs were disabled walking is lame. I told my father. Just then the trolleybus came. My father didn't get on the trolleybus. but ran immediately to chase the man back instead. And said sorry to him. It showed me my father's passion and kindness. It also showed me that we should consider each other's feelings.

2.   I went to buy cigarettes for my father. The boss of the shop let me take them by myself. At night, the street lamp was very dark, and I

bought it in a hurry and then climbed up the mountain slope to go home (houses in Chongqing are mostly built on the mountain slope).

When I got home and found there is an extra cigarette. My father said to me very seriously : At any time, don't take advantage of small things. "Stealing needles as a child, grow up to steal" gold." send the extra cigarette back immediately. At that time, I was less than six years old and felt wronged. I had to send the cigarette back at dark night.

When I grew up, I deeply realized that this is a father's love, he is teaching me to be a man, to be honest from an early age not take any advantage. I will remember my father's teaching forever.

Later my father gave up his habit of smoking with a strong will before his grandchild was born.

There was another quote from my father that stuck in my mind.

He often said to me: A man will meet many difficulties in his life. When it happened, you can touch your *Laok*e (Sichuan dialect of head,). Oh! the *Laoke* is still there, no problem! There will be hope!! Encourage me when encountering big things, as long as the head is still there, it's no problem, there is still hope!!

Now, "Oh! the *Laoke* is still there, no problem!" has become a classic sentence of the Taijiquan class. My Taijiquan students have learned the sentence

Father's open-minded, optimistic, challenging and fearless attitude towards life, let me benefit for life! I'm a lucky one with a mentor-like father for navigation.

Since then, whether in work, marriage, or interpersonal relationships, I have kept my father's teachings in mind and followed his example in everything, so my life is still smooth and complete. I even got a doctor's degree (Doctorate in Acupuncture and Oriental Medicine) at the age of 70.

I learned from my father, I have been promoting Taijiquan for more than 40 years.

The new book 《108 Stories of Taijiquan Healing》, will be published soon. I think it is the best gift to comfort my father!

Father is an ordinary man. However, his enthusiasm, kindness, and unremitting promotion of Taijiquan has won great respect. Hundreds of people visited my father's memorial service after he died in the USA: an elegant lady came to my house to plant tulips to show nostalgia; a mother and her daughter send flowers on his memorial day every year. At a memorial service in Chongqing, thousands of people played Taijiquan to commemorate him! Thus, respect and love do not depend on a person's power or money. He is dead, but he lives in our hearts forever.

My father was incorruptible and poor all his life, leaving no property to his children, and even some debts, but he left us the most precious wealth - Taijiquan and noble qualities, and the principles of life!

在 1930 年，我的父亲患有肺结核咯血（当时还没有治愈这种疾病的药物）。父亲便随绍兴国术馆长曾寿昌先生学习太极拳。他每天修练太极拳，竟然不用药就治愈了他的肺结核。

从那时起，他就开始志愿教太极拳，已经有 67 年了。他希望世界之人都能练太极拳，享受太极拳带来的美好生活。父亲说这是他一生的理想和责任！父亲是太极拳传播者，他的学生普及在重庆，北京，和广州市。不仅如此，父亲还把太极之花传播到了美国。许多美国学生甚至开车 7 到 8 个小时向他学习。他从年轻到年老，从未停止过教太极拳。父亲说，只要他还活着，他就永远不会停止教太极拳，直到他去见上帝。这种执着，这种大爱，让我们深深地受教育。

父亲教导我们习武要先修德，太极拳是一具有文化内涵的文明拳种。他告诫我们：善良、乐观、宽容、坚毅、勤奋、好学、热诚、尊师爱友，仁义是太极拳精神。道德好拳才能打的好。父亲还要求我们兄妹远离酒色财气，学会感恩，滴水之恩当涌泉相报。做一个正直的人。每天他都要写日记反省自己有无不当之处？坚持读书练字没有？他的言行，激励着我们，甚至他的开怀大笑，也深深地影响着我们，我们三兄妹也都养成了咧咀大笑的习惯。

有两件小事让我于身难忘：

一次，我与父亲在等电车，有个人来问路，父亲告诉他，他要去的地方不太远，可以走过去，不用等车，于是问路人走了。后来我发现那人腿有残疾，走路是瘸的，便告诉了父亲。这时电车来了，但是父亲没上车，而是立即跑步将那个人追了回来，还搀扶着他说对不起⋯⋯。

这件事让我看到父亲的热诚、善良，还让我知道做事待人要考虑对方的感受。

还有一次，我去给父亲买烟。卖烟的老板让我自己拿，晚上路灯很暗，我急忙买了就爬大坡往家里赶(重庆的房子多建在坡上)。回家一看多了一支烟，父亲很严肃地对我说："马上还回去，任何时候都不能占小便宜。小时偷针，长大偷金。那时我还不满6岁，感到很委屈，漆黑的夜晚还得一个人将那烟送回去。长大后我才深深地体会到这是父爱，他在教我做人，从小就要诚实不占任何小便宜。我会永远记住父亲的教导。

后来父亲在孙子辈出生之前，用坚强的意志戒掉了几十年抽烟的习惯。

父亲还有一段话也让我铭记在心。他常常对我说："人的一生会遇到很多的困难。遇到困难时，你就摸摸脑壳(四川话脑袋)，哦！脑壳还在，没问题！"。勉励我即是遇到天大的事，只要头还在，就没问题，就有希望！！

现在这段话已经成了太极拳班的经典之句，我的太极拳学生，都学会了"摸脑壳，没问题"这句话。父亲的豁达，乐观，接受挑战的大无畏的人生态度，让我终身受益！

我是一个幸运儿，有导师般的父亲指导。此后无论是工作、婚姻、人际关系，我牢记父亲的教诲，事事以父亲为榜样，故自己的人生尚顺利、完满。甚至在 70 岁古稀之年，还获得了中医博士学位。我还向父亲学习，无论在国内国外也坚持推广太极拳 40 多年。

新书《108 个太极拳健身者的故事》即将出版，我想这是告慰父亲在天之灵的最好的礼物！

父亲是一个普通的老百姓。但是他的热情、善良，坚持不懈的推广太极拳，赢得了人们极大的尊敬。父亲在美国去世后有数百人前来悼念：有个优雅女士专门来我家门前种上郁金香以示怀念；一对母女每到他去世的日子就寄鲜花来；在重庆的追悼会上有上千人打太极拳纪念他！可见尊敬和热爱绝不是依人的权势、钱财而定。他虽已去世，却永远活在了我们的心中。

父亲一生清贫，没有给儿女留下任何财产，甚至还欠了点债务。但是他却给我们留下了最宝贵的财富—太极拳与高贵的品质，及做人的准则！

106. Memory of my Grandfather
回忆我的爷爷

By Jian Chuan

My grandfather is a sincere person with great integrity. I often reflect on moments of him, feeling like it was just yesterday.

My grandfather respected teachers and valued education. Once his son (my uncle) visited him in Chongqing from Hangzhou, grandpa took him to revisit uncle's high school teacher and showed respect by presenting the teacher with a Chinese painting, saying "always appreciated your teaching". This impressed me and showed me how we should appreciate our teachers.

Grandpa considers reading/writing/study as the most important thing in his life, I often reflect on the image of his office with a tremendous amount of books/papers, feather pens, and the smell of inks, and ink stones. This is part of the reason why I love reading as I grow up.

Grandpa had high respect from their community. I often lived in grandpa's house at weekends. Wherever we go, people always greeted them with: "Morning, Master He, thank you." This is because grandpa taught Taijiquan (free of charge) at parks to lots of people, their enthusiasm and knowledge of Taijiquan helped many people, physically and psychologically. When the instruction is in progress, all people are quiet and are concentrated on following the steps of my grandpa. I am very proud of my grandpa.

Grandpa often visited me at my high school and brings me food and snacks. He sometimes watched me from the window, he is consistently amazed that all the students were studying diligently without making a single noise. He is very proud that his grandson was one of them with a promising future.

Grandpa is a sincere person who gives all he has to his family, his wife, children, and grandkids. He never spends extravagantly; always cooks at home to save money, always lives a simple and humble lifestyle. The only time I saw him dine at a restaurant was one day he served as judge for a Taijiquan competition at a downtown gym, far from home, after that long and exhaustive day, he was afraid that I may be too hungry and took me to the nearest restaurant to feed me. That is the first and only time I saw grandpa dinned in and of course, that meal to me is the most delicious and becomes my precious memory of my grandpa.

In my first year in college, Wuhan is far from grandpa's home (Chongqing), grandpa had an exciting travel plan with his Huangpu Military classmates, which was going over the first stop would be Wuhan that meant grandpa can visit me again. my classmates all want to see him, a real person from that famous military Academy, though many of them were surprised that grandpa did not look like a graduate from a military academy, but rather looked like a scholar.

After my college, I worked in Nanjing, grandpa visited my mom and me many times, I had a chance to show him around, and visited many temples. I listened to grandpa's whispering on calligraphy, Tablet Carving, Buddhist Scripture, ShenDao, and benefit a lot, full of interest. I also had a chance to treat him with vegetarian food from several famous temples. This is a great honor to me.

When I pursue my graduate studies in Honolulu, Hawaii, grandpa visit me on my first Christmas, again it was my greatest honor to show him around, sightseeing most of the Island of Oahu by bus (I didn't have a car at that time), Pearl Harbor, China Town, a Chinese church where grandpa had a photo with Mr. Zhang Xueliang and his wife Ms. Zhao Si. As. a soldier, grandpa admired General Zhang's patriotic enthusiasm，I witnessed the excitement of the meeting，and leave them with precious group photos.

Grandpa is a sincere person with great integrity; has been a loving husband and father, he lives a simple and ordinary life, he has respect for every person who knows him, and he is a real model for all of his children and grandchildren. This is why I miss him, why I love him the most, and why I respect him as a great man.

I am so proud to be his grandson. Writing here, my tears can not help flow without end! I can not control myself. I will miss him and love him forever

I want to try my best to be a person with great love like grandpa!

我的祖父是一个非常真诚、颇有气节的人。我经常回忆他，感觉就在昨天。

我的祖父尊重老师，重视教育。有一次，他的儿子（我的叔叔）从杭州到重庆看他。爷爷带他去看望叔叔的高中老师，爷爷和舅舅合写了一个条幅，"不忘师恩"送给当年的老师，给幼小的我留下深刻的印象，也告诉我应该如何尊敬我们的老师。

爷爷一向把读书、写字、学习看作是他生命中最重要的事。家里满柜子的书，书桌上墨水，宣纸，毛笔，砚台，让我从小闻到笔墨的香味。这也是我成长后喜欢阅读的原因之一。

爷爷受到了他们社区的高度尊敬。我经常在周末住在爷爷的家里。无论我们走到哪里，人们总是向他打招呼："早上好，何老师，谢谢你。"这是因为爷爷在公园里教很多人太极拳（免费），他对太极拳的热情和知识对很多人在身体上和心理上都有帮助！在教太极拳时，人们鸦雀无声，紧随爷爷的脚步。我为我的爷爷感到非常骄傲！

爷爷经常去我的高中看望我，给我带来食物和零食。他有时看我上晚自习，他总是惊讶于所有的学生都在努力学习，没有发出任何噪音。他很自豪，他的孙子是他们中前途光明的人之一。

爷爷是一个真诚的人，他为他的妻子、孩子和孙子奉献了一切。他从不铺张浪费；为了省钱总是在家做饭，过着简单朴素的生活。我唯一一次看到他在餐馆吃饭，是在有一天，他在市中心担任太极拳比赛的裁判，离家很远。经过漫长而疲惫的一天后，他又担心我太饿，便带我到了最近的餐馆。这是我第一次也是唯一一次与爷爷在餐馆吃饭。当然那顿饭对我来说是最美味的，也成为我对爷爷的珍贵记忆。

在我上大学的第一年，武汉远离爷爷的家（重庆），爷爷和他的黄埔军校同学有一个令人兴奋的旅行计划。第一站便是武汉，这意味着爷爷可以再来看我了。我的同学都想看他，一个来自著名的军事学校的真人，尽管他们中的很多人都很惊讶爷爷看起来不像军校的毕业生，而是像一个学者。

大学毕业后，我在南京工作，爷爷去看我妈妈和我很多次。我有机会带他四处走走，参观了很多寺庙。我听爷爷低声讲解书法，碑刻，佛经，禅道，受益匪浅，兴趣盎然。我也有机会用著名寺庙的素食来招待他，这对我来说是一件非常荣幸的事。

当我在夏威夷的檀香山继续我的研究生学业时，爷爷在我的第一个圣诞节第一次来看我。我很荣幸地带他参观，乘巴士游览了瓦胡岛的大部分地区（当时我没有车）中国城，珍珠港，在一个中国教堂，爷爷与张学良先生和他的夫人赵四小姐合了影。同为军人，爷爷敬佩张将军的爱国热情，我见证了他们会面时的激动心情，并为他们拍下珍贵的合影照片。

爷爷是一个真诚正直的人，也是一个好丈夫和慈爱的父亲，他过着简单而平凡的生活。他得到了每个认识他的人的尊敬，他是他的子孙后代的真正榜样。这就是为什么我想念他，为什么我最爱他，为什么我尊重他 —— 这个伟人。

我很自豪能成为他的孙子。我会永远想念他，永远爱着他。写到此处，我不禁泪水长流！不能自己。

我要努力成为一个像爷爷这样有大爱的人！

107. In Memory of my Grandpa
缅怀我的外公

by Hai Hai

Since I can remember, Grandpa has always been the most respectable and amiable family member around me.

He is a soldier of iron blood. As a graduate of Whampoa Military Academy, he has always had the unique temperament of a soldier. No matter where he goes, he always stands tall and straight, with high spirits and shining eyes. Until late in his life, his love for the country and the family were always strong as before. He loves to watch TV broadcasts and ongoing political and social news, especially news reports on Taiwan and cross-strait relations. Although sometimes, like other old people, he may doze off while sitting in front of the TV and watching for quite a long time. After a short pause, he will soon wake up full of energy and continue watching attentively. His house is often crowded with visitors and friends. He likes to discuss with them various issues including national events such as the disintegration of the Soviet Union and the development of Sino-US relations. They can always have heated exchanges and debates.

He is an old man but has ardent love for his daily life. In the 1980s and 1990s in China, people have just solved the basic problems of food and clothing. There was no internet or social media, highways or private cars. But even looking back from today's perspective, Grandpa's late life was so rich and colorful. He has visited many famous sites in the country, and also traveled across the oceans several times. When I was a child, I liked to repeatedly read over the photo booklets of his traveling, from which I learn more about the outside world.

He loves playing Taijiquan. An authentic descendant of Yang Style Taijiquan with the military experience he is, Taijiquan is the backbone of his body and the most shining aura on him. He keeps practicing from Taijiquan, Taiji sword, Taiji broad sword, to Taiji hand-pushing every day, boxing, no matter whether it rains or shines. In his own words, he would stop only practicing during long-distance traveling by air. Even when sometimes he travels by train, as long as he stops halfway, he will get off the train and do some practicing on the empty platform for a while, attracting everyone to watch.

He also loves teaching Tai Chi. From Chongqing to Beijing, from China to the United States, he will teach wherever he goes. His movements of Taijiquan look rather relaxed and elegant, reinforced by his white hair, healthy figure, and ruddy complexion, always attracting many fans of different ages and nationalities over the years. Mr. Ken, my college foreign teacher, is also one of them. The first time he gave us an English class, he asked where we could learn Tai Chi. I immediately recommended him to Grandpa, and Grandpa agreed with no hesitation. In order to learn Tai Chi, Ken rushed from school to Grandpa's place every morning before dawn. With the help of Grandpa's hand-by-hand instruction and my efforts of translation, he really managed to learn the full 118 movements of Yang Style Tai Chi boxing.

One day, when I stood in a woods in Beijing , gesturing to review the Taijiquan movement following the descriptions in the Taijiquan book written by Grandpa. A passing middle-aged man saw the picture of Grandpa on the cover and told me excitedly that he himself also had the opportunity to learn Taijiquani from this old man.

After years of practicing Taijiquan, Grandpa has an excellent physique that ordinary people can't match. As long as you get close to him and touch his shoulders or arms, you can feel exactly a sort of internal power in his body, which was usually described as the top master in those traditional novels of martial arts. Every piece of his practice movement is full of energy, smooth, and couple hardness, and softness.

There is a story that I've heard from Grandpa many times. A security guard in his workplace is a graduate of the police school and a master of wrestling and combat. He looked down upon Taijiquan, which looks so slow and useless. One day he challenged Grandpa and said that if Grandpa defeated him, he would worship him as his Taijiquan Master. On the day of the challenge, more than 200 people gathered around the playground of the workplace to see the contest. There seems to be a great disparity between a thin old man and a tall and big young guy. All of sudden, the young man rush to Grandpa quickly to attack him. Grandpa stood still and when the young man approached, he separated his fists with the Taijiquan movement named 'Part the Wild Horse's Mane on Both Side', pushed him back six or seven meters and then drag him down with another Taijiquan movement and won easily. The young man admitted his defeat and immediately bowed down to Grandpa as the master. On the same day, many onlookers admired Grandpa's Taijiquan skills and chose to follow as his students.

On another occasion, Grandpa took me to catch the bus. At that time I was already in college. After waiting for a long time, the bus finally came and was already full. The people waiting for the bus rushed up, squeezing against the bus door. The middle of the carriage is still relatively empty, but the people, either those who just got on the bus or those about to get off later, all stuck at the door and couldn't move. They were reluctant to move and shouted loud to those below who were still waiting to get on, 'Impossible to get on, don't squeeze anymore'! I also suggested Grandpa wait for the next one. But always elegant as he is, he suddenly grabbed the door handle with a big step and shouted, "Why don't you let us get on? The middle of the carriage is still empty, so let's move in together!" While hugging the people in his front and making a powerful movement, he not only managed to step onto the bus together with a bunch of people ahead of him, but also squeezed out some room for me. He then turned around, saying 'Come on' and pulled me onto the bus. The people in the front had been pushed by him to east and west. I could hear a lady complaining, "Why is this old Granny so strong?" I started sniggering, with a Chinese saying floating in my mind, 'This is Chinese Kung fu!'

He is a warm-hearted old man. He has many friends and students, which brings him not only quite social resources but also lots of requests for help from time to time. In those days there was no phone, let alone a cell phone or WeChat. Most of the communication were carried out through personal visit and face-to-face discussion. So I still remember that Grandpa was often not at home, running all around for the various matters of relatives and friends. One day, an elderly relative was seriously ill and needed surgery as soon as possible, but it was difficult for him to make a treatment appointment due to a lack of access to the reliable hospital. He entrusted me to ask Grandpa for help. When I went to find him at home at noon, he had just returned from outside after a busy morning, and I could see that he was very tired. But when hearing about my request, without saying any word, the old man took a quick nap and went out to catch the bus, so as to visit his student who worked in a famous local hospital. He didn't come back until that evening. Then he told me that everything had been arranged and the elderly relative may go directly to that hospital and see his student for medical treatment the next day.

Meanwhile, he is also a frank and lovely old man. In his later years, it is difficult not to be 'ordinary'. He may also 'show off' from time to time. He likes to share with others his experience of long-term practice of Taijiquan. Like other parents, he also loves to talk about the various achievements of his children. His son and daughters are all successful in their careers, and all of his four grandchildren went to famous universities. In order to make him happy, the family members may report to him all kinds of progress and good news either in careers or in school. While feeling happiness and pride, he is always eager to share these good news with his friends or neighbors, which often embarrassed his family members who want to keep a low profile.

Grandpa has been a chivalrous and upright man all his life. He has been strict with himself, always keeping personal integrity, refraining from smoking or alcohol, and hates to bother others. Even on that last night in the United States, his sudden but forever departure was in his sleep. Without any toss and pain or any disturbance to the family at all, he left us so resolutely and decisively, just like his whole life, simple, pure and clear-cut as always. I felt lucky that I happened to be in the States at that time, for I could drive, after hearing the sad news, for more than six hours overnight to see him off for the last time.

Now Grandpa has been away from us for more than 20 years. But when I recall everything about him, they were as fresh as yesterday. His love for life, love for his family, as well as his integrity, kindness, and self-discipline have always been his most admirable and unforgettable qualities of him to me. 'The best way to memorize someone is to inherit his spirit and follow his example'. So I wrote down these fragments of my life to remember my grandpa, and encourage myself to be a man like him.

从我记事的时候起，外公始于就是我身边最可敬也最可亲的亲人。他是一位铁血军人。作为一名黄辅军校的毕业生，他身上一直有着军人的独特气质，不论走到哪里，他都身肢挺拔，精神矍铄，目光如炬。直到晚年，那份家国情怀，也都始于浓烈如初。他爱看新闻联播和时政要闻，特别是对有关台湾情况和两岸关系新闻报道，总是听得聚精会神。虽然有时也像其他老人一样，在电视机前坐久了，看着看着就打上盹了，不过稍息片刻，他就很快满血复活。他的家里常常人来人往，高朋满坐，他也很喜欢和客人们侃侃而谈，包括像苏东剧变和中美关系这样的国家大事，他们总能进行热烈的讨论交流。

他是一位热爱生活的老人。二十世纪八九十年代的中国，人们刚刚解决基本温饱问题，没有互联网和社交网络，也没有高速路和自驾车。但从今天的视角来回看，外公的晚年生活却是丰富多彩，充实无比。他走过祖国的千山万水，也曾几度飘洋过海。小时候我就很喜欢反复欣赏他家里的照片册子，从他在各地的留影中去更多地了解外面的世界。

他喜欢打太极拳，作为杨式太极拳正宗传人和军校出身的他，太极拳是他的立身之本，也是他身上最闪耀的光环。刀剑拳、太极推手，他日日坚持，风雨无阻，用他自己的话说，只有坐飞机时才会不打。即便坐火车旅行，只要中途经停，他都会下车在空旷的站台上打上一阵，引来众人围观。

他也喜欢教太极拳。从重庆到北京，从中国到美国，他走到哪里，就教到哪里。鹤发童颜、气色红润的他，打起拳来行云流水，飘逸舒展，本身就是自带流量的广告，多年来吸引了众多不同年龄、不同国籍的粉丝。我的大学外教 Ken 也是其中一位。他给我们第一次上英语课时，就询问大家在哪可以学太极拳。我立即向外公推荐了他，外公也欣然同意。为了学拳，Ken 每天早上天不亮就从学校赶到外公每天的练拳地点，在外公手把手的教学和我努力地"翻译＋陪练"的相助之下，还真就学完了杨式 118 式太极拳。

还有一次，我在北京的一个树林里，对着外公写的太极拳书，比划着温习太极拳招式。一位路过的中年男子看到封面上爷爷的照片，很兴奋地告诉我，他自己也跟这位老人学过太极拳。

多年习武的他，确实有着常人不及的过硬体质。只要和他一近身，一搭手，就能感觉他身上有着武侠小说里那种顶尖高手的浑厚内力，不仅一招一式，能量满满，而且刚柔并济，绵绵不绝。

我听外公讲过多次。他们单位一个保安人员，毕业警察学校，格斗擒拿样样在行。他不大看得起太极拳，认为慢慢吞吞没有用。一次，他向外公发起挑战，称如果外公打败他，他就学习太极拳。比武那天，200多号人围在单位大操场观看。一个瘦老头对一个高高大大的年轻人，貌似悬殊很大。只见那人快速猛冲向外公，外公稳稳的站着不动，待其攻来，用一招野马分棕将其拳头分开后，向他发力一推，让他倒退了六七米远，后来又用一招履法将其摔倒，轻松获胜。此人甘拜下风，立刻拜外公为师父，当天，不少围观者纷纷折服外公的太极拳功力，当即也向外公拜师学艺。

还有一次，外公带着已上大学的我去赶公交车。等了好久，车终于来了，已然满载，而候车的人们一拥而上，更是把车门挤得死死的。其实车厢中间还比较空，但刚上车的、一会要下的人都卡在门口那，无法动弹。车上那些不愿费劲再挪动的人就纷纷向下面想上车的人喊着："上不来了，别挤啦！"我也想和外公说等下辆吧。可一贯儒雅的他突然急了，一个剑步抓住车门把手，一边大声嚷着："凭什么你们上了就不让我们上了？车厢中间还空着呢，大家一起往里挤挤！"，一边拥着前边的人一发力，使劲往里一挤。愣是不仅把一堆人连同自己都挤上了车，还给我挤出一个空位，回头一把拉着我，"快上来！"我赶紧上车后，发现前面的人已然被他挤得东倒西歪，哎哟连天。一个女士还在抱怨，"这老头这么大岁数了，怎么还这么大劲？"我心里直偷着乐，脑海里飘过四个字"孔武有力"。

他是一位古道热肠的老人。他朋友多，学生多，使得他既拥有一定的社会资源，也让他时常遇到来自亲朋好友的各种各样的求助。那个时候没有电话，更没有微信，凡事都需要登门走访联络，所以印象中他经常不在家，为了亲朋好友的事情四处奔波。一次，一位亲戚家老人患重病需做手术，但求治无门，委托我找外公帮忙。我中午去家里找他时，他刚从外面忙了一上午回来，看得出很疲惫，但一听说此事，二话没说，小憩了一会就出去赶公交车，找他在医院工作的学生去了。直到傍晚才回来，告诉我都已安排妥当，亲戚第二天就可以去找他学生办理入院了。

他也是一位率真可爱的老人。即到晚年，也难以免俗，时时会有些"凡尔赛"，喜欢与别人分享自己长年锻炼的受益心得，也会像别的父母一样，有意无意地介绍子孙们的成就。他的子女们都事业有成，几个孙子也都是名牌大学，为了让他开心，家人们不时向他汇报工作上、学习上的各种进步和好消息，他每次高兴之余，却也总是迫不及待地与去别人分享，常让想低调的家人们哭笑不得。

外公一生对人行侠仗义，对己严格自律，洁身自好，烟酒不沾，更从不爱麻烦别人。直至那晚他在美国的突然离去，也是在睡梦当中，"嘎嘣脆"地一般，毅然绝然地与我们告别，自身没有经历任何折腾和痛苦，也没有对亲人丝毫牵绊和拖累。正如他的一生，清清爽爽，干净利落。我庆幸当时正好在美国，得以闻讯后连夜驱车六个多小时赶到那里，见了外公最后一面，为他老人家送行。

外公离开我们已经二十多年了。但回忆起他的一切，依然记忆犹新，往事如昨。他对生活的热爱，对家人的关爱，还有他的正直、善良和自律，始于是让我最为敬佩、也最为难忘的道德品质。"最好的缅怀是传承"。所以我记录下这些生活片断，缅怀我的外公，也以此自勉，努力做一个像他那样的人。

108. In Memory of my Grandfather
纪念我的爷爷

By He Yunsha

Hawaii, the silver pearl in the Pacific Ocean, is renowned for its beautiful sunlight, white sandy beaches, dreamy blue water, and the Hula Kahiko dance. Located in Hawaii's capital, Honolulu, there was a house unlike any others, not because of its grandeur or its serenity, not because of intricate architecture or historical significance, but because it holds a special meaning in my heart.

A handsome gentleman used to live in this house. He is a political legend who has changed the history of China. He is the son of the Grand Duchy of China's the Mandurian States. His story, of his loyalty and rebellion against Chiang Kai-shek, of his struggles against the Japanese invasion during World War II. The tragedy of losing freedom from the young age of thirty-six, including the stories of his and his wife was also spread for a while. It was also spread for a while. They were a mirror reflecting the stories of an entire generation.

His name is Peter Plat Chang (Zhang Xueliang).

However, this general and his legacy are not the reason this home is so special in my heart. For within this house, a picture hangs on the wall. Within this picture, the general sat, wrinkles etched on his face, like tree rings displaying the difficulties and hardships of his life.

This photo (Fig.7) is not the reason either. For behind the general, a younger gentleman stood, an infectious smile on his face and a witty glint in his eyes, with a very infectious smile He was my grandfather, his surname is He, his given name is Ming, and his other given name is Jingzhi.

Because I have never seen my own grandfather, so I called him the grandfather.

Since I was a child, I knew that my grandfather lived far away in Chongqing. In my impression, the first time I see him is about four years old, grandfather tall and handsome, with a body like iron, and he walks like a tiger.

At that time, I was watching the Hong Kong drama warrior Huo Yuanjia, knowing that my grandfather was a martial arts expert, I really admire it.

In the 1980s, when my grandfather first taught Taijiquan in the courtyard for the first time with hundreds of students, I also ran up to him to show signs and felt very brave.

At that time, there was no Internet, no movies, not even square dance, and Taijiquan became a way of life. In the courtyard hundreds learn Taijiquan, their aim is physical fitness, plus chat with one an other.

Later, when grandfather began to teach Taiji knife, Taiji sword, it was really a sword light and knife shining and everyone is busy making sword or knife.

I still remember one of the inscriptions on a student's sword: "Oh master's skill and thy student sword; wield it and thou would hear my word."

As I grew older, simple childish hero worship toward Grandfather turned into intellectual curiosity. What kind of person was he? How did he turn out to be such a man of stature? Not only was he a Kungfu master, but he was also a great artist and poet. He had taught Taijiquan and other

300

forms of Kungfu to tens of thousands of students for many decades, yet he never charged a penny. Why would he do such a thing? What kind of past brought him to become who he was? Through endless inquiries to families and friends, I began to piece together the puzzle, watching a legend's story happen right before my eyes.

My grandfather came from an official family. Since Ming Dynasty, there were many Jinshi (a ranked scholars). Although the family was down, some people were small officials like county officials in Qing Dynasty.

Born as the son of an official in the Qing Dynasty, my grandfather enjoyed a relatively peaceful upbringing. While barely seeing his father and raised mostly by his mother and relatives, he enjoyed a wistful life in a village, with stories of cats and parrots filling his childhood. When he grew up, he moved to Shaoxing, a small yet important city in southern China near the Yangtze River, and became an advisor of the city's governor. This year is a turning point in his life.

Every morning at 6 o'clock am, Grandfather, who at that time was merely 20 years old, would run up Kuaiji mountain (a tiny mountain, filled with trees, streams, mist, and historical legends), until he reached a flat intersection, where he would practice Taijiquan for hours.

Every morning, grandfather was dressed in white and stepped up on the Kuaiji Mountain. In the woods, surrounded by streams, mist, winding countless historical legends of the hills, practicing boxing, day after day. His white robe, focused expression, elegant and powerful movements, attracted many audiences. Seeing his face focused in intense concentration, many people would stop and watch. They called him the "White Crane Master."

On a slightly cold winter day, while my grandfather was practicing taijiquan a middle-aged rich merchant who often traveled between

Shaoxing and Shanghai, approached him, and inquired about his family, who taught him Taijiquan, and what was he doing.

My grandfather told him that he used to suffer from tuberculosis, so he decided to learn martial arts. He has learned from a lot of masters and learned many boxing, but finally, he studied from the Taijiquan master Zeng Shouchang, (curator of Shaoxing Martial Arts, who is a good friend of Yang Chengfu, Master of Yang Style Taijiquan) and finally cured his lung disease without Medicine. His current position within the government is the advisor of Shaoxing county magistrate.

Grandfather is not only proficient in martial arts, but also a poet, a young man with a dream. He soon became a friend to the merchant, and met the merchant's daughter, a young girl who was proficient in arts and literature, and soon began their love story that would last for half a century.

Shaoxing was a small place but has many outstanding people. It is the homeland of Goujian (King of Yue, who lost his kingdom through inhuman suffering and sacrifices, so as to strengthen his power and restored his kingdom at last), and the burial site of great Yu (who saved China from the Great Flood) in ancient China, and the home town of Qiu Jin martyrs in the modern era.

On July 7, 1937, the Anti-Japanese War broke out in China. Full of blood grandpa, leave his fiancee for Wuhan without hesitation, to join Whampoa Military Academy (see 16th alumni record of Whampoa Military Academy). After he graduated from Whampoa Military Academy, he was appointed as an instructor at this academy.

During anti-Japanese aggression war, nearly four million Chinese soldiers were killed, while ten times more civilians than soldiers perished.

On August 13, 1937, the Japanese aggressors attacked Shanghai, and broke the dream of Grandpa and the daughter of the rich merchant. It was the darkest days in the twentieth century in China.

Before long, his family's silk shop, her parents, family, and villa were all in the flames of war turned to dust and ashes. After her villa was bombed and her parents lost in the ensuing fire, the daughter of the rich merchant decided to wipe away her tears and leave Shanghai for Chengdu to find her true love.

Those were dark and confusing times; all historical artifacts and records of her travel were lost. What little evidence we had about this journey was her personal integrity and her recount of certain events that took place in China.

We knew she searched in the dark in the war-torn land for two years. She roamed through landmine-filled farmlands, hid in rivers filled with dead bodies, ghosted her way through battlefields red with blood stain, and was stricken with serious diseases and almost died in a snowstorm night for months. She evaded soldiers, gangsters, and murders, but also met people with simple decency to spare her with a hot meal. In the end, perhaps through insane luck or a herculean iron will, she persevered.

At that time, grandfather was an instructor of the Whampoa Military Academy in Chengdu.

One day, when he was training his soldiers in camp, a soldier reported: "There's a lady outside the barracks and she wants to see you, sir."

Grandfather walked outside of the barracks and saw no lady, but a poor little person waving at him enthusiastically, in the shaggiest clothing that seemed to be stitched from multiple fabrics. No matter what the colors were those fabrics, they were now just blackish grey covered in soot and dirt. Grandfather was stunned for what seemed like an eternity or a few minutes, then he ran towards her, lifted her up in the air and told her that they will be together forever. Grandfather told me, on that day, at that moment, the woman was radiating with light. The afterglow of the entire sky fell onto her cloth, and made it the most beautiful and divine. Perhaps, that's the only time I saw tears well up in Grandfather's eyes in my life. Now that I have grown up and thinking about this, Chengdu was the city where Grandfather met his love for life, and it was a city devoid of sun, how could it have an entire sky of afterglow? But at that moment, Grandfather probably thought the beauty of the entire world belonged to her, my grandmother.

Yes, in a fairy tale, the prince will marry the princess and they would live happily ever after. In reality, at least in Grandfather's life, he had spent a wonderful time with Grandmother for a while. But in those warring decades, even the most beautiful dream would not have lasted long. After the World War II ended, China continued to fight for a few years and finally received a much-deserved peace. At this time, Grandmother with three children passed away due to all the illnesses she had endured during her journey to find him. Her youngest daughter, who was six at that time, grew up in the military, went through a cultural revolution, and became a living legend as well. By the way, she also happens to be my mother.

As for my grandfather, after experiencing the loss of his wife, he is still open-minded.

After Liberation, he went through various movements smoothly, finally ushered in the era of reform and opening up. At this time, my 60-year-old grandfather began to glow with vitality in Chongqing and ushered in another peak of life.

After retiring from the army, and when China finally ended the cultural revolution, he started to devote all his energy to Taijiquan. He traveled far and wide, and taught tens of thousands of people in Chongqing and Beijing. Even though he lived on a measly small retirement salary, he never charged a penny for his Taijiquan lessons.

In 1995, Grandfather traveled to the Minnesota United States. And I still remember, at the University of Minnesota, the giant hall was filled with people of all stripes, colors, beliefs and party affiliations. But all of them gathered for a common cause, that is to witness the wonder of an old Kungfu Master and learn from him the near-mythical wonders about Taijiquan. After seeing how Grandfather in his 70s, throw off a two hundred pounds guy, they cheered and became faithful students in way of Taijiquan.

Ten years later, Grandfather passed away in a peaceful sleep. Throughout his entire life of war and of love, he's never been sick. Even in his passing, he was still a strong man with tremendous physical and mental strength. Comparing him to the general who took a photo with him, I have to say, even though Grandfather received far less fame than the general, he too touched tens of thousands of people, helping them through difficult times and becoming strong. Even though he never become rich with money, he was content and lived a bountiful life.

The general once commented that he had not truly lived after the age of 36 due to his perpetual imprisonment, but Grandfather lived through war and peace, had multiple children and grandchildren, and many students. I still remember a remembrance speech made by a dear friend named Adam during Grandfather's funeral. "Master not only taught me Taijiquan, kept my body healthy, he also showed me how to maintain an optimistic mind in the highest state possible through good times and bad times." His optimism, smile and courage warm the people around him.

Grandfather's life was full of ups and downs, but no matter what he faced, he remained optimistic, loyal, loving, caring, happy, and open-minded. Sometimes, when I look at the child of my own, I could feel Grandfather's smile shone through their brilliant smiles too.

305

在宽阔的太平洋上，有一串珍珠般的岛屿，夏威夷。说到这里，一般人想到的是明媚的阳光，洁白的沙滩，梦幻般碧蓝的海水，以及热情奔放的草裙舞；在夏威夷的首都，檀香山市内，坐落着一座别有意义的住宅。它的特别，不在于他的庄严和美丽，不在于它精巧的设计与历史的底蕴，它的意义仅仅深藏于我心中。

这里曾经居住着一位英俊的老人。他是东北王的独子。他的故事，他对蒋介石的忠诚和反抗，他对日本入侵时的挣扎和抵抗。他三十六岁后失去自由的的悲剧，包括他和他夫人的故事，也曾轰传一时。他的功过一生，是那一代人的缩影。

他的名字叫张学良。但是，这位将军的故事和传奇并不是让我觉得这座房子有特别意义的原因。因为在这房子里，墙上挂着一幅照片。（见附录图7）在这张照片里，你会看到将军坐在那里，一脸的皱纹如同树轮一般，记载着他一生的困苦。

但这张照片依然不是让我对这房子充满感情的原因。如你仔细看去，少帅的身后有一位"年轻"很多，眼神敏锐的老人，带着非常有感染力的微笑。这位老人，姓何，名明，字镜之，是我的外公。

因为我没见过亲爷爷，所以我管外公叫爷爷。

从小时候，就知道远在重庆，住着一个爷爷。印象里第一次见他是四岁左右，爷爷高大英俊，身体像铁打的，走起路来虎虎生风。那时候正在看港剧大侠霍元甲，知悉爷爷是武术大行家，真的是佩服得五体投地。

在1980年，爷爷第一次在大院里教太极拳，学拳者甚多。自己也跑到他身边比划来去，觉得自己神勇极了。那时没有网络，没有电影，连广场舞都没有，太极拳变成了一种生活之道。大院里好几百人来学拳，图的就是个强身健体，外加交际聊天。

后来爷爷开始教太极刀、太极剑的时候，那可真是剑光霍霍，刀光闪闪。一时间人人奔走，买刀造剑的不知凡几。大院里舞刀弄枪的气氛浓厚一时，青龙剑，桃木剑，纸片剑层出不穷。现今依然记得，有位学生赠爷爷双股剑，上面用小凯毛笔题诗，诗曰："师传剑术徒造剑，握剑练剑如吾面"。

慢慢长大了，对爷爷单纯的崇拜，变成了一种好奇的探究。这样一个老人，不但武艺高强，而且运笔如刀，书法天成。他先后授徒上万，却一直分文未取。他究竟有着什么样的过去，有着怎样的经历？在向父母亲人不断的追问中，渐渐拼出了这样一个传奇的人生。

爷爷出身于官宦世家。祖上自明朝起，就多出进士。而在清朝年间，虽说家道中落，也有人做县官这样的芝麻小吏。到了爷爷这一代，他的父亲一直在外地当知县。自己在农村的家中倒是过的清净悠闲，养着八哥，养着小黑猫，属于家道不好不坏，读书识字，四书五经不少的最后一代满清知识分子的后代。爷爷弱冠之年来到了绍兴，做起了绍兴师爷。这一年是他的人生转折。

每日清晨，爷爷一袭白衣，蹬上会稽山。在树林密布，溪水环绕，薄雾轻袭，缠绕着无数历史传说的小山中练拳，无一日间断。他白色的长袍，专注的神情，优雅而充满力量的动作，吸引了许多观众。看到他那全神贯注的样子，大家开始称他为白鹤大师。

在一个微寒的冬日，爷爷正在练拳，一位中年儒雅，经常在上海绍兴走动的富商叫住他并问他师承何人，在绍兴有何公干。

那时的爷爷患有肺结核，所以下定决心学武健体。他拜过的师傅很多，学过的拳法也不少，但是最后师从太极拳大师曾寿昌，（绍兴国术馆长，太极拳大师杨澄甫的好朋友）也算是名门高徒，最终也治好了自己的肺病。

爷爷不但武艺精通，同时还是一个诗人，一个有梦想的年轻人。在一练一聊的过程中，爷爷和中年富商结下了友情，并结识了他的千金，展开了一场惊心动魄的琼瑶式爱情。

绍兴，地虽不大，人杰地灵。古有治水之大禹之陵墓，卧薪尝胆终于复国之勾践，近有侠女秋瑾义士。所以这里的人，可不是什么"不知秦与汉"的村民，而是出没于商路航线的商人和勇敢的战士。

1937年7月7日，抗日战争全面爆发。满腔热血的爷爷，义无反顾地离开了他的未婚妻，投笔从戎，到武汉黄埔军校参军（见黄埔军校 16 期同学录）。

1937 年 8 月 13 日，日寇进攻上海，打碎了爷爷和富商千金的琼瑶梦。一时间，旧的生活随风而去，新的腥风血雨已经来临。那是二十世纪最黑暗的日子，近四百万中国士兵战死，几乎十倍的老百姓彻底消失在神州大地。

不久，她家的绸缎庄、她的父母、家人和别墅，都在熊熊的战火之中化为灰烬。在她失去了父母后，终于要走出富贵门，在这场前所未有的浩劫中，踏出自己入世的第一步。

我不知道，不能想象，这样一位不食人间烟火的千金，是如何在战火缤纷的大地上，寻找她的未婚夫的。她到底遇过什么，经历过什么，如何在烽火遍地中找到了自己的未婚夫，已经随着老人家的早逝而不可考。但我知道，这位娇娇小姐在险恶的战火中走了整整两年。

这期间，她穿过地雷密布的田间，在尸体漂流的水中躲藏过，在染满鲜血的战场上潜行，也生过大病，差点死在风雪夜中。

她很智慧的躲开士兵，土匪，恶霸，但也碰上过不少好人，能分给她一顿热饭，让她在寻寻觅觅中得以一线的喘息。有一点我们非常肯定，她离开上海时，是位不食人间烟火的千金；当她到达成都的黄埔军校时，已经是一位身体极度羸弱，但意志却比钢铁还要坚强的女性。

一天，当时爷爷正操练炮兵，忽然听说有人来找，怀着无穷的疑惑，他来到了校门口，看到一个娇小的身躯，裹在一身不知道什么颜色的破棉袄中，对他挥着手。他愣住了，足足一个世纪那么长远，也可能只有几分钟，然后他飞快的跑过去，一把抱起前面的伊人，告诉她今生今世，两人的心永远在一起。爷爷说，那时候漫天的彩霞，都落在了这个女人的身上，那身破棉袄，焕发出了无比美丽的光彩。可能，这是我唯一一次看到爷爷落泪。现在长大了，想了想，其实成都那么多阴天，素有蜀犬吠日之说，哪有什么漫天的彩霞。但是我想，那时候的爷爷，一定觉得世界上所有的光彩都只属于奶奶一个人。

在童话中，王子与公主的结局总是美好的。在现实中，至少在爷爷的生命中，再和奶奶重逢，的确过了一段美好的时光。但是在那样一个兵锋激荡的大时代，就算是最美的梦也是要醒的。二战结束后，中国又打了几年，终于来到了和平年代，而这时，有了三个孩子的奶奶，终于因为常年的病痛，在三女儿年幼时就撒手而去。而这位自幼丧母的三女儿，在军队中长大，在支边中成长，后来也变成了一个颇有传奇色彩的女性，也就是我的母亲。至于我的爷爷，在经历过丧妻之痛后，依然能够豁达。他顺利地度过了解放后的多次运动，迎来了改革开放的年代。

这时，60岁的爷爷在重庆开始焕发的活力，迎来了生活的另一个高峰。在重庆，北京，他都广收门徒，打拳授业，好不热闹。但有一点，那时候的他，虽然只有几十块钱退休金，却从来不收费。门徒上万，完全没有想过要收个拜师费。这一教，就到了1995年。在国门打开的时候，爷爷的拳法也教到了美国。至今我还记得，在美国明尼苏达大学里，一大厅黑压压的人，什么肤色的都有，什么发型都有，所有人来这里只有一个目的，目睹一下中国来的功夫老人，看他是怎么一巴掌轰飞一个两百斤的壮汉。不消说，爷爷又有了大批的美国学徒。

爷爷在美国去世时，没有任何痛苦，一晚安静的睡去，就再没醒来。一生戎马的他，自从治好肺结核后，一直无病无痛，直至去世，依然身体健康硬朗。相比张学良将军，虽然爷爷的名气几乎没有，但是却也触动了成千上万的人，让他们都能够健康平安。虽然一生清贫，却豁达自知。少帅曾感叹，自己36岁后就没有了人生。可爷爷的人生几起几伏，终究能够化险为夷，一生自由自在，子孙满堂，学生遍天下。现在犹记得一个外国友人给爷爷的献词，他说："何先生不仅仅教会了我如何打拳，如何保证身体的健康，更让我认识到如何在人生的挫折中，永远保持最最乐观心绪和积极的态度。"

他的乐观，微笑和勇气，始终温暖着周边的人。

爷爷一生的坎坷，以及永远满腔热血，永远乐于助人，永远用最积极乐观的态度看待人生的性格，深深地落在了我们每一个后代的血液中。有时候，我看着自己的女儿们快乐的面对困难，一恍惚，就会看到爷爷的阳光的笑容。

M   The Health and Fitness Benefits of Taijiquan
太极拳的养生健身效果

The Health and Fitness Benefits of Taijiquan 太极拳的养生健身效果

By Dr. Luis Jin Lei

Taijiquan is truly a timeless medical art and health exercise encompassing all of the mind, body and spirit. Originating in ancient China, it is one of the most effective exercises to maintain human health and wellness. Although known as art with great depth of knowledge and skill, it can be quickly learned and eventually mastered by consistent practice and fully harness its vast health and fitness benefits, often lasting for a lifetime. Because of its abundant health effects, cultural origin, sports characteristics, martial arts connotations, rhythmic aesthetics, social entertainment, philosophical thoughts and other strong Chinese elements, Taijiquan is beloved by hundreds of thousands of practitioners and enthusiasts around the globe. At the same time, as the essence of the Chinese traditional culture, it is respected by people of different nationalities, races, genders and ages in the world. Therefore, based on the sheer number of people who love and practice this type of exercise and its wide influence, it certainly qualifies as number one frequently practiced exercises in the world, bar none. Thus, to date, the health and fitness benefits of Taijiquan are well-documented and verified by a large number of modern research studies (many of which are by prestigious institutions like Harvard and Yale Universities), so now let's re-visit and re-examine what some of these main benefits of practicing Taijiquan actually are!

太极拳是真正一门囊括了思想、身体和精神的永恒医学艺术与养生运动。它起源于古代的中国，是维护人类健康的最有效的运动之一。尽管它是一门知识和技能都很深奥的艺术，但它可以很容易地学会，练习者在每天练习后不久就开始受益，而很多人在持久练习后会享用一生。由于太极拳的养生效果、文化渊源、运动特点、武术内涵、韵律审美、交际娱乐、哲学思想等浓厚的中华文化因素，它深受全球数十万练习者和爱好者的喜爱。同时，又作为中国传统文化的精粹，为世界不同民族、不同种族，不同性别，不同年龄的人所尊崇。因此，依据喜爱、参与此项运动的人数和其广泛的影响力，被誉为：世界第一运动。因此，迄今为止，太极拳的健康和保健作用已被大量的现代研究报告所证实（许多是由类似哈佛大学和耶鲁大学等著名机构进行的），现在让我们再来回顾一下练习太极拳的这些好处究竟是什么吧！

(1) Improves Memory Performance 增加记忆力

Under the normal human aging process, like anything going through years of grind, our memory will eventually fade over time. Whilst some people remain vigilant in seeking the fountain of youth via a "silver bullet" type of pill or some form of diet or supplement, practicing Taijiquan has shown clinically to improve short and long-term memory. This may be because Taijiquan includes training in sustained attentional focus, shifting, and multi-tasking which could help train memory, concentration, and the overall cognitive function. Once Taijiquan is learnt, please don't forget to practice it every day, and when you do, the mind becomes sharper and more reactive, and allows more memory to be retained. By practicing Taijiquan consistently for some time, you may gradually feel full body relaxation and stronger mind power.

在人类正常的衰老过程中，就像任何东西经过岁月磨练一样，人们的记忆力最于会随着时日的消逝而减退。虽然我们中的有些人仍然刻意地寻求可以一颗可以永驻青春之泉的"银弹"药片，饮食或保健品，但练习太极拳在临床上的确显示可以有效改善短期和长期记忆。究其主要原因是可能太极拳包括持续注意力集中、转移和多任务的训练，这可以帮助训练记忆力、注意力、与整体认知性功能。一旦学会了太极拳，请不要忘记每天练习，当你这样做的时候，头脑会逐渐变得更敏锐，使记忆力日增月益，再通过坚持练习太极拳一段时间后，你可能还会逐渐感到身体全部放松及较充沛的脑力。

(2) Unblock and dredge the meridians (channels and collaterals) to circulate the qi（vital energy）and xue (blood), move the blood to improve the cardiac functions 畅通经络气血，加快血液循环，强心

Once the body and mind become disarrayed, restlessness, skin or muscular disorders arise. If the meridians (channels and collaterals) are blocked or congested, then quite possibly the *qi* (vital energy) and *xue* (blood) are not getting through smoothly, when the *qi* becomes stagnant and/or the blood becomes stuck, people are more prone to be ill. This is where Taijiquan shines as it can help dredge the meridians to circulate the *qi* and *xue* once again. Nowadays, with the fast-paced lifestyle in general society, most people who live and work in the larger metropolitan areas are extremely busy with daily work and life, so often cannot find free time or a quiet place to properly exercise. Taijiquan is a simple and gentle exercise, requiring little time, almost no equipment and little space to practice. When practiced, it can enhance the cardiac functions, so that the pulse becomes slower, steadier and stronger. Medical science has shown that Taijiquan can also enhance the elasticity of blood vessels and reduce the possibility of blood vessel rupture. For an office-type worker who sits in front of a computer or is always on the phone at the office desk) for an extensive amount of time doing work, neglecting the postures often will result in muscle stiffness, tightness and soreness around the spine, neck, shoulders and other parts of the body. Sometimes the skin will even have breakouts of acne or carbuncles, in fact, most of these muscular, skin, physical and mental diseases almost always are stemmed from the disharmony of the *qi* and blood, caused by the clogged *qi* and *xue* in the meridians. Generally, through a prolonged period of Taijiquan practice, the *qi* and *xue* will become gradually smooth again, while the body and mind will be brought back to a state of balance or (unified into one). Furthermore, according to Traditional Chinese Medicine principles, myocardial infarction is mostly due to blood stasis, or caused by the blockage of blood vessels by blood clots. A steady diet of Taijiquan practice can reduce the formation of such blood clots and reduce the possibility of such myocardial infarction.

　　一旦身体和心灵变得混乱，就会出现烦躁不安、皮肤或肌肉紊乱。如果经络和脉络不通，那样人体血液一般就不再通畅了，血液如不通畅，人就容易得病，而练习太极拳能够帮助人打通经络，增强人体血液循环与新陈代谢。现代城市人大多工作生活繁忙，导致经常没有时间或没有地方去专门运动，而练习太极拳时，也无需大空间与锻炼器材，它是一种柔和运动，能增强心脏功能，使心脏慢而有力。太极拳能增强血管弹性，减少血管破裂的可能性，长期在办公室坐着办公，时间一久没注意姿势，肌肉僵硬了，全身还时常会出现小疙瘩或皮疹，其实这些肌体皮肤或身心疾病如（身心不和，身心不安，身心不平等）大多来自于气血不通，气血不通的原因一般是经络不通导致，所以，一般通过一段时间太极拳练习，气血逐渐通畅了，身心也就合一了。而且，练习太极拳还可以预防心肌梗塞，中医认为心肌梗塞主要是气血不通畅，血凝块堵塞血管而造成的，太极拳能减少血凝块的形成，减少心肌梗塞的可能性。

(3) Relaxing the pulse 放松脉搏

When the meridians are blocked, the pulses naturally become taut, resulting in the whole body becoming tense and stiff. If you begin to practice Taijiquan for at least half an hour every day or practice until the palms are slightly sweaty, you will eventually see the whole body gradually become relaxed.

经络不通，脉搏自然僵硬，全身都很紧张，很僵硬，如果每天练太极拳至少半个小时，或者练到手心微微出汗，全身就会开始放松了。

(4) Increasing muscle strength 增强肌肉力量

Whenever there is an irregular lifestyle, such as poor eating and sleeping habits, they may often lead to poor health status, resulting in stiff muscles throughout the body, less flexibility, feeling weak and lethargic throughout the day. By practicing Taijiquan, muscle strength will gradually be restored, and not only will the sinews, tendons and bones become stronger, but various joints will also become more flexible.

生活没有规律，如不良的饮食和睡眠习惯，极易导致全身肌肉僵硬而没有弹性，就是没有力量，通过太极拳之后增强肌肉力量，还有强健腿力和足力、筋骨，而且关节也会变得灵活起来。

(5) Reduce the overall disease of the five zang (viscera) and six fu (bowls) 减少五脏六腑疾病

The five *zang* (viscera) and six (bowls) need exercise, if they do not exercise, they will naturally be hardened and may be prone to be ill, therefore, the gentle movement of Taijiquan is more suitable. It can enhance the secretion function of the digestive glands, promote regular peristalsis of the stomach and intestines, increase appetite, enhance the function of the elasticity of the internal organs, to prevent or delay many organ-specific diseases as we age.

五脏六腑需要运动，如果不运动，自然就硬化而得病，因此，柔和运动的太极拳比较合适。可以增强消化腺的分泌功能，促进胃肠有规律的蠕动，增加食欲，增强五脏六腑弹性的功能，可以预防或延迟随着年龄而来的很多脏腑性疾病。

(6) Prevent or treat the "three highs" and obesity 防治三高与肥胖

The dread three words, "you have three highs" - high blood pressure, high blood sugar/h glucose (diabetes), and high cholesterol, often haunt people worldwide. If you've been diagnosed with one or more three highs, and have tried all types of medications to little or no effect, it is wise to immediately begin to learn Taijiquan, then practice for a few months to see if you can lose some of that stubborn extra weight, and perhaps the "three highs" will be "magically" leveled off. Taijiquan is usually good at preventing or reducing high blood pressure, diabetes and cholesterol along with controlling obesity, habitual constipation and other chronic diseases.

有三高，医生们开了很多药方，没有大的效果，开始太极拳吧，现练上几个月，看看是否有减肥的效果，说不定三高就开始三和了。临床与科研都显示，太极拳对于防治高血压、糖尿病、肥胖症、高血脂、习惯性便秘症等慢性病都有良好的作用。

(7) Keeping the spirit joyful! 保持精神快乐！

Medical science often postulates that regular practice of Taijiquan will eliminate ischemic symptoms of the heart or lower blood pressure. Making the body reduce fatigue, soothe the mind, and relieve panics and palpitations. It is said that human emotions (spirit) and wisdom have a close relationship with the nature of the blood. Taijiquan can also help to reduce blood sugar and lipids, eliminate blood stagnation and blood-related disorders and remove other toxic waste in the blood, and when there is no more toxic waste in the blood, the *qi* and *xue* will flow smoothly and the spirit will be joyful once again.

医学讲，定期坚持练习太极拳，会消除心脏缺血性症状或降低血压。使人体消除疲劳，精神愉快，缓解心慌心悸。人不愉快和智慧与血液的本质有关系，太极拳能减少血糖，血脂；排除血淤，血里的垃圾，血里少了垃圾，气血通畅，人精神会愉快很多。

(8) Maintaining lustrous skin, youthful and beautiful shape 保持体形与皮肤年轻美丽

The beauty of a person (skin and shape) is also directly related to the nature of our blood. When there is no more toxic waste in the blood, the person's skin tone and shape naturally become more beautiful. Practicing Taijiquan can help reduce the toxic waste in the blood, rid of the accumulated fat, and help maintain the lustrous skin tone and beautiful shape.

人的皮肤美不美与血液性质，有直接关系。血里没有垃圾，人一定漂亮、美丽，血里垃圾多，人自然就不漂亮。因此，太极拳能排除体内的垃圾和血里的垃圾，减少人体腹部脂肪的积聚，保持人体的形体美。

(9) Stronger kidney function 强壮肾功能

When people are lazy at exercising such as being reluctant to move, or sitting for a long time, all can contribute to negatively impacting the kidneys, and may result in various kidney deficiencies, nephritis, kidney stones, and other kidney dysfunctions, etc. When the kidney blood supply becomes insufficient, when that happens, the liver blood becomes insufficient; when liver blood is insufficient, the heart blood becomes insufficient, and people start to get sick easily. In order to get better, people often take medications, which increase the burden on the kidneys. Practicing Taijiquan can help reduce the need to take medications, thus enhancing the functions of the kidneys naturally.

人如果比较懒惰，不愿意活动，或坐的时间长，都可能伤害肾，造成肾虚，肾炎，肾结石，肾功能退缩，因此，肾供血不足，肝血就不足；肝血不足，心血就不足，就开始生病了。为了治病吃药.，增加肾的负担，练习太极拳能减少吃药，从而自然地增强肾的功能。

(10) Improved brain clarity when studying 在学习时提高大脑清晰力

When one stays in front of the computer or studies (reads or writes) for an extensive period of time, the brain will become fogged and bogged down. If doing a quick round of Taijiquan during a break, one can receive some fresh air, helping recharge and revive tired brain cells, removing mental fatigue, this will surely improve one's overall learning process and make studying more efficient.

当人长时间待在电脑前，学习（看书，写字），大脑会变得不清晰，这时练习太极拳几分钟，接受新鲜空气，大脑思维活动会变得清晰了、灵活了，消除了大脑的疲劳，提高了学习的效率。

(11) Sharper vision and mind power 增强视力与脑力

When reading books, playing computer games, or swiping Wechat too much, one's vision will degrade over time. According to the relevant studies by experts, when practicing Taijiquan at least three times a week, each time minimum for an hour, and continuous practice for four months.

When compared with people who do not exercise, the former group had a sharper vision, with an increased memory and reaction time than the latter group.

看书，打电脑游戏，发微信过多，视力退化了，据有关专家测试，每周太极拳三次，每次一小时，连续坚持4个月者与不喜欢运动的人相比，前者反映敏锐，视觉与记忆力均占优势。

(12) Life-span Extension 益寿延年

People who live past the age of ninety-five (longevity people) remain rare in today's world, and some studies have shown that most longevity people practice at least one or two hours of Taijiquan a day. Indeed, life-span extension lies in motion, and Taijiquan as a form of ancient fitness with moderate movement and stillness intertwined like a yin-yang fish may help relieve neuromuscular tensions and stabilize emotions so that life-span can be naturally extended.

在世界上活到九十五岁的人（长寿人）是很稀少的，有研究显示，大多数长寿的人都每天最少要练上一两小时。的确，生命在于运动，而太极拳是一种静中有动、动中有静的健身方式，可以缓解神经肌肉紧张，稳定情绪，这样寿命自然延长。

(13) Symmetrical exercises to compensate for the body's acquired deficiencies 对称运动，弥补人体后天不足

During daily life and work, people either intentionally or unintentionally formed a number of habitual stereotypes. Most if not all of these habitual movements are mostly one-way-based movements. For example, the upper limb movement in daily life is generally led more with the right hand; lower limb movement is more led by a moving right foot; upper middle movement is also more led with the right shoulder.

The opposite is true for left-handed people. Whether left or right, they are always one-way movements. These types of one-way movements, over time, will cause the central nerve of the brain to weaken the reverse regulation function, which will inevitably lead to an imbalance in the internal functions of the human body, so the diseases occurring on a single lateral side are indeed common. In ancient China, there is a common saying that "male left female right". The movement structure of Taijiquan emphasizes the right first if the aim is the left, the bottom first if the aim is the top; when the force is applied, the front is split and the back is supported, and the top is withered and the bottom is stepped on. The upper and lower parts of the body are unified in opposition and integrated. Thus, it effectively strengthens the reverse regulation function of the brain, maintains the overall coordination and balanced development of human movement, and overcomes the defect of one-way movement causing diseases.

人们在日常生活、工作中，有意或无意地形成了诸多习惯定势。凡是习惯动作多属单向偏颇运动。如日常生活中上肢运动一般多用右手；下肢运动多以右足发力；中上盘运动也多用右肩。左撇子反之。无论是左还是右，均系单向运动。这种外形的单向运动，天长日久，使大脑中枢神经减弱了逆向调节功能，由此势必导致人体内部机能左右失衡，故人体患病多集于一侧确为常见，有"男左女右"的俗话。太极拳的造型结构，强调欲左先右、欲上先下；发力时，讲求前吐后撑、上枯下踩。周身上下对立统一、浑然一体。从而，有效地强化了大脑的逆向调节功能，保持了人体运动的整体协调与平衡发展，克服了单向运动致病的缺陷。

The above 13 benefits are what's known of Taijiquan so far, what people might not realize is that a healthy body is generally supported by three types of exercise. The first type of exercise is aerobic exercise, which can increase cardiopulmonary and cardiovascular functions, but also can consume the body's extra protein. All aerobic exercises shall be done under a relaxed state, such as slow walking, gentle hiking, Taijiquan, floating in a swimming pool, etc, the premise of aerobic exercise is to exercise in a relaxed state. The second type of exercise is called limb elongation, where the flexibility and health of your body joints, muscles, tendons and ligaments come into play. Some of these are needed for body elongation exercises, when the person is older, the ligaments and joints begin to contract inward, the back becomes hunched, the waist is also bowed, so we must do joint elongation exercises, and such exercises are a prerequisite for maintaining the body joint flexibility and stability. The third type of exercise is to do instant anaerobic exercise, note that these are not continuous anaerobic exercises, which actually stimulate your muscles to increase functions. Again, do not do continuous anaerobic exercises, as such exercises will make your muscles too tight resulting in thickened muscle fiber density, in fact, it is a kind of damage to the muscle. Doing instant anaerobic exercise is a very short time to muscle tension stimulation so that you can enhance muscle function, but also avoid damage to muscle fibers. Of course, there are people that only focus on one exercise, such as sitting meditation, as they were told sitting meditation is a kind of relaxation-based aerobic exercise. But it does not have any aerobic movement of the limbs, limb elongation, or instant anaerobic exercise. So over time, as people sit for a long time, their joints often will have problems, even with some muscles atrophied; There are also people who prefer to do muscle training, those who like to train specific parts of their body, such as making their legs and arms to become very thick. So the muscle may look good aesthetically but actually, those thickened muscle fibers are damaged; Thus one shall not be partial to just a single exercise, all three exercises need to be taken. Do you know what exercise is the perfect combination of these three exercises? It's a no-brainer, Taijiquan is the only one.

　　以上列举的练习太极拳 13 个好处是目前已知的的情况，大家可能不知道是一个健康的身体一般是由三种运动方式来支撑的。第一种运动方式就是有氧运动，有氧运动可以增加心肺功能，心血管功能，还可以消耗人体的蛋白质，所有的有氧运动都是处在放松状态下进行的，如慢走、散步、太极拳、在水里漂浮游泳等 ... 有氧运动的前提就是在放松状态下运动。第二种运动方式是叫肢体伸长运动，身体关节的柔韧度，肌肉，肌健、韧带这一些是需要做身体的伸长运动，当人老的时候，韧带、关节就开始往里收缩，收缩以后背也驼了，腰也弓了，所以一定要做关节伸长运动，保持做肢体伸长运动是保持身体关节柔韧度灵活度的一个前提。第三种运动方式就是要做瞬间的无氧运动，不是做持续的无氧运动，无氧运动是刺激你的肌肉，保持肌肉的功能。不要做持续的无氧运动，长时间的无氧运动就把肌肉练的很硬，肌肉的纤维密度就增粗了，实际上是对肌肉的一种损害；瞬间的无氧运动是时间很短对肌肉紧张的刺激，这样既可以增强肌肉功能，又能够避免对肌肉纤维的损害，这就叫瞬间的无氧运动。我们经常看到有一些人只注重一项运动，如有的人喜欢打坐，都说打坐是一种放松有氧运动，但他没有肢体的运动，没有肢体的放长运动，没有快速的无氧运动，所以很多人坐久了关节都有问题，肌肉都萎缩；也有的人专门练肌肉，那些把腿胳膊练得很粗，然后肌肉练得很丰满，实际上看起来肌肉很丰满好看的样子，实际上他的肌肉纤维增粗已经受损害了；所以说不能偏重那一项，要三种运动要结合起来；那么什么运动能把这三种运动完美的结合起来呢，是太极拳。

　　Why Taijiquan? First of all, it is a relaxation-based exercise. When we practice Taijiquan, the body becomes very relaxed. Remember, the Taijiquan instructor's first lesson is always about relaxation. Relaxation is one of the important characteristics of taijiquan; second, taijiquan is a stretching exercise. It is called "stretching the tendons and pulling the bones, connecting the bones and tendon," and the instructors always say that all the movements are done in an elongated state; third, Taijiquan is an instant anaerobic exercise. Taijiquan is a combination of rigidity and flexibility, with hammering, push-hands and fisting, all of which are instant anaerobic exercises; so it is said that Taijiquan can perfectly combine these three exercises together, which is why many practitioners feel good after practicing Taijiquan and feel that their health is changing for the best, because Taijiquan combines all three exercises perfectly in unison.

为什么是太极拳，首先，太极拳它是一项放松运动，我们练太极拳身上都很放松，太极拳老师一上课了都讲放松，放松是太极拳的重要特性之一；第二，太极拳是一项伸长运动。叫撑筋拔骨，接骨枓榫，练拳时候老师都讲，所有的动作都是在伸长的状态下完成的；第三，太极拳是瞬间无氧运动。太极拳刚柔相济，有炮锤发劲推手搏击，这些都是瞬间的无氧运动；所以说太极拳能把这三种运动完美的结合在一起，这就是我们很多人练了太极拳以后感觉自己身体很舒服，觉得健康状况在改变，原因就是因为太极拳把这三种运动完美的结合起来了。

It is often said that society is people-driven; then what about people, how are they driven? Actually, people are health-driven; health is a vitality, health is productivity, and you have nothing without health. The body can be thought of as a health bank, and we have to deposit money into this bank every day. We also use the money in the health bank every day, so if you do not save money in this bank, you might end up with an empty account, with no money left after the overdraft, the bodily health will be severely discounted. So we need to save money for our health bank every day, and practicing Taijiquan is the best way to save that health money

Everyone should learn taijiquan and practice it every day. Taijiquan is not only a form of exercise, but also a culture and a spirit; that's why 2008 practitioners showcased it at the 2008 Beijing Olympics, and the theme of that one scene was called 'nature'. There is no one who is not touched by this display of group Taijiquan, which represents the spirit of Chinese people, so learning Taijiquan is not only one way to train your body, but also an inheritance of Chinese culture. At the same time, we should reflect a noble moral spirit in our practice of Taijiquan, and influence people around you with a healthy body and mind, so that not only you are healthy yourself, but you also bring health and happiness to your family and friends.

人们常说社会是以人为本；那么人以什么为本呢，人以健康为本；健康就是生命力，健康就是生产力，你没有健康就什么也没有。身体是一个健康银行，我们每天都要向这个银行存钱。我们现在每天都在用健康银行的钱，不存钱用到最后你就没钱了，没钱以后就透支了，透支以后身体就打折了。所以说我们每天要向自己的健康这个银行存钱，打太极拳就是最好的健康存钱方式。

大家都应该学习太极拳，都应该多练习太极拳，太极拳不仅仅是一种运动方式，更是一种文化，同时是一种精神；所以北京奥运会上用2008个人来展示太极拳，那一个场景的主题就叫自然。没有一个人不被这场太极拳所感动的，他代表了中国人的一种精神，那么学习太极拳，不但可以把自己身体练好，也是对中华民族文化的继承，如果你喜欢中国文化，你会打太极拳就是对中华民族文化的继承与传承。同时我们应该在太极拳练习中要体现出一种高尚的道德精神，用一个健康的身体、健康的心态去影响你周围的人，不但你自己健康同时也给你的家人，你的朋友带来健康，带来快乐。

The biggest difference between Taijiquan and other forms of exercise is that it is a kind of movement that uses intention but not force, it emphasizes intention but also emphasizes form, and guides the physical body with mindfulness. Taijiquan is a movement of the whole body, with the intention of guiding the *qi* (vital energy), and all the changes in forms, one move and one style are all about the intention in the body first, the intention of moving the body, and the intention of settling the form. It is because of this *Kung Fu* characteristic of Taijiquan that even in their old age, the old martial artists who are experts of *Kung Fu* are not deaf, nor blind, nor sunken feet, and have a higher skin tone or sensitivity than normal people much younger than themselves. So while practicing Taijiquan, it is more important to create a harmonious self. All happiness and joy are built on the premise that we are healthy and can have some sense of well-being and happy life, to pass this mentality to people all around us, so that we can all live a better, healthier and wiser life. So don't wait, for a healthy and happy life, for you and your loved ones, start learning and practicing Taijiquan today!

太极拳与其他拳种的最大区别，就在于它是一种用意不用力、重意也重形、以意念支配肉体的运动。太极拳行功走架，全神贯注，以意导气，所有外形变化，一招一式无不讲求意在身先，意动身随，意静形止。正是由于太极拳的这一功法特点，功深艺高的老拳师即使到了晚年，也多是耳不聋、眼不花、脚不沉，其肌肤的敏感性仍异于常人。所以在练好太极拳的同时，更重要的是要营造一个和谐的自我。一切所有的幸福和快乐都建立在我们健康的前提下，能够对自己健康快乐的生活能有一些感悟，能够把这种心态传递给自己周边的人，让我们的生活更加美好、健康和智慧。为了健康快乐的生活，开始练太极拳吧！

Note：Dr Louis Lei Jin, DAOM, is a NCCAOM board certified and state licensed acupuncturist in Wisconsin, USA. Having served as a past president of Wisconsin Society of Acupuncturists, USA, Dr. Jin is currently the director of membership of American Traditional Chinese Medicine Association (ATCMA) and secretary general of its academic subcommittee of Medical Taiji and Qigong. Besides, he is also the current director of affairs of the Chinese Medicine Luobing Society of America. Additionally, Dr. Jin serves as an overseas board member of multiple specialty academic subcommittees of the World Federation of Chinese Medicine Societies, including the External Treatment Methods in Oncology, the Endocrinology, the Internal Medicine, State-Target Strategy, the Anti-Aging, etc. (All the part-time jobs are volunteer work）

金雷 美国针灸与东方医学博士，全美 NCCAOM 认证与威州执照针灸师，原威州针灸师学会会长，现任全美中医药学会 ATCMA 会员部部长兼医学气功太极专业委员会秘书长，美国络病学会总务部部长，世界中医药联合会肿瘤外治法专业委员会，内分泌专业委员会，内科专业委员会，态靶辩治专业委员会，抗衰老专业委员会海外理事。所有的兼职全是做义工。

Appendix 附录

1. Picture 照片

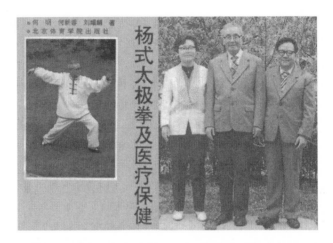

Fig.1. Cover of 《Yang Style Taijiquan & Health Care》 & its . Authors of this book He Xinrong, He Ming, Liu Yaolin《杨式太极拳及医疗保健》作者：左起何新蓉、何明、刘耀麟

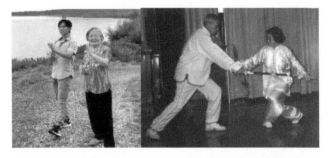

Fig.2 The Authors of this Book
Steven Yang & He Xinrong
本书编著者阳思达与何新蓉

Fig.3 Master He Ming and his daughter
He Xinrong perform Taiji Sword
何明与其女儿何新蓉表演太极对剑

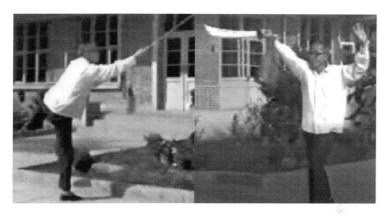

Fig.4. Master He Ming performs Taiji Sword and Broad Sword 何明大师表演
太极剑和太极刀

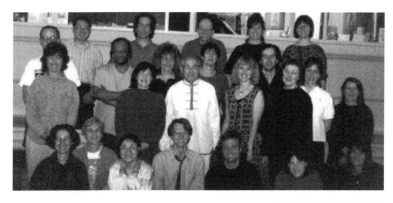

Fig.5 Master He Ming and his American students 何明大师与美国学生

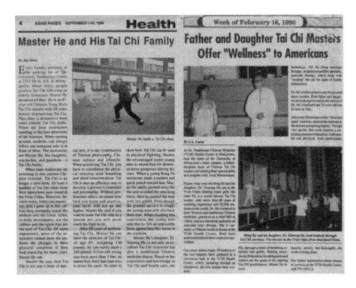

Fig.6《Master He Ming and his Tai Chi Family》《何明大师和他的太极之家》

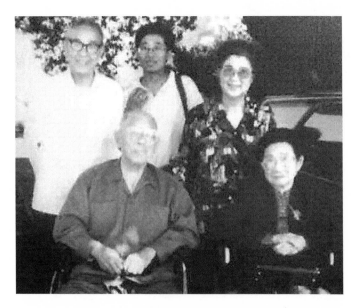

Fig.7 General Peter Plat Chang & his wife Edith zhao (1ˢᵗ row) & He Ming (2ⁿᵈrow left), in Honolulu 张学良将军与夫人赵一荻（前排）与何明（后排左1）合影于檀香山

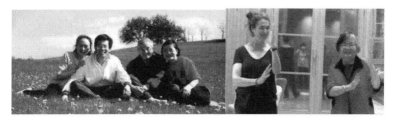

Fig.8: Liu Wei, Gong Changzhen and
Ming &He xinrong in Minnesota
刘伟 巩昌镇夫妇与 何明 何新蓉父女
在明州

Fig.9 Da Xiao & He Xinrong He
Practicing Taijiquan in a
Brazil Hall 大笑与何新蓉
在巴西大厅练拳

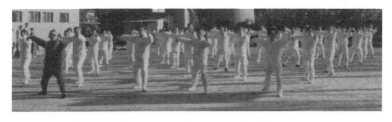

Fig.10. Students of He Ming perform Taijiquan in Beijing 何明与学生在北京表演太极拳

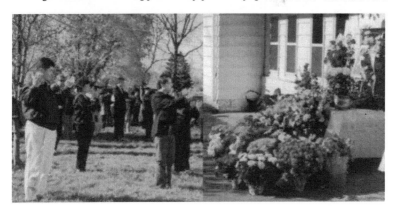

Fig.11. His students perform Taijiquan at the Memorial Ceremony for Master
He Ming in Minnesota 在明尼苏达举办的何明大师追思会上，学生们表演太极拳

331

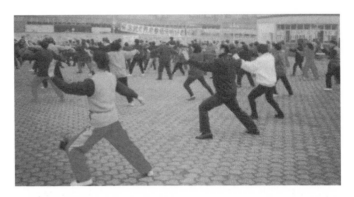

Fig.12 Miss the good old martial arts boxer He Ming (Chongqing) 怀念武术界
老拳师何明好老师（重庆）

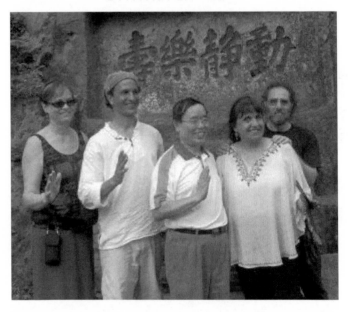

Fig.13. Kay(left 1).Cary (left 2) ,Esther and her husband(left 4.5) and He family in
Shaoxing Fushan

Kay, Cary， Esther 等与何氏家人在何明当年练太极的绍兴府山

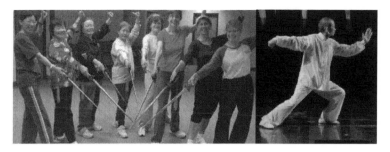

Fig.14. He Murong (second left) & her students   Fig.15.Professor Zou Zhen

are playing Taijii Sword 何慕蓉（左 2）   is playing Tijiquan

与她的学生表演太极剑   邹溱教授在明州表演太极拳

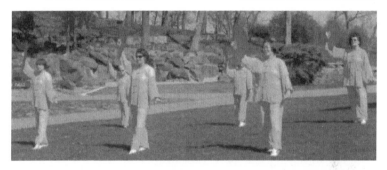

Figure 16. Friends are performing Taijii Fan 拳友们表演太极扇

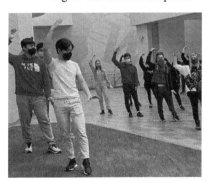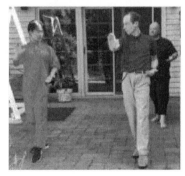

Fig.17-18 The Author of this book Steven Yang is teaching Taijiquan

阳思达在教太极拳

333

2. Bibliography 参考文献

[1] [ADAA (Anxiety and Depression Association of America). About ADAA Facts & Statistics Updated August 2017. https://adaa.org/about-adaa/press-room/facts-statistics]

[2] Practicing Tai Chi can reduce the saliva cortisol content. After practicing Tai Chi for 18 weeks, the researchers at Coburg University, Germany found significant (p<0.05) reductions of saliva cortisol (post and follow-up), which seems to be an indicator of general stress reduction. [Esch T, Duckstein J , Welke J , Braun V. (Division of Integrative Health Promotion, Coburg University of Applied Sciences, Coburg, Germany. esch@hs-coburg.de) Mind/body techniques for physiological and psychological stress reduction: stress management via Tai Chi training - a pilot study. Med Sci Monit。 2007 年 11 月 ; 13 （11）: CR488-49

[3] (UQ revitalises ancient art of Tai Chi to help people SMILE 14 May 2015 Share link: http://tinyurl.com/pqj7mvs)

[4] [WANG guo-pu et al. The changes of brain wave characteristics and state-trait anxiety of different state-trait anxiety sufferers before and after doing Tai Chi exercise. 《Journal of Physical Education》 2006-06
http://en.cnki.com.cn/Article_en/CJFDTotal-TYXK200606011.htm]

[5]Association of Tai Chi exercise with physical and neurocognitive functions, frailty, quality of life and mortality in older adults: Singapore Longitudinal Ageing Study By Shuen Yee Lee, Ma Shwe Zin Nyunt, Qi Gao, Xinyi Gwee, Denise Qian Ling Chua, Keng Bee Yap, Shiou Liang Wee, Tze Pin Ng. [Age and Ageing, Volume 51, Issue 4, April 2022]
afac086,https://doi.org/10.1093/ageing/afac086

Published:05 April 2022

[6] Tai Chi improves psychoemotional state, cognition, and motor learning in older adults during the COVID-19 pandemic

April 2021Experimental Gerontology150(1):111363

DOI:10.1016/j.exger.2021.111363

Made in the USA
Monee, IL
29 September 2023

43667204R00208